Born in 1960, former Salvation Army trombonist Kitty Churchill is a freelance journalist who writes mainly about sex. She lives in London with her husband and a selection of novelty rubber goods.

THINKING
OF
ENGLAND

A CONSUMER GUIDE TO
SEX IN A COLD CLIMATE

Kitty Churchill

An *Abacus* Book

First published in Great Britain in 1995
by Little, Brown and Company

This edition published in 1996 by Abacus

A CIP catalogue record for this book
is available from the British Library.

ISBN 0 349 10864 1

Typeset by M Rules in New Baskerville
Printed and bound in Great Britain by
Clays Ltd, St Ives

Abacus
A Division of
Little, Brown and Company (UK)
Brettenham House
Lancaster Place
London WC2E 7EN

To Davey and Ian

Acknowledgements

I would like to thank Alan Samson and Jo O'Neill at Little, Brown and my agent Jane Turnbull for overriding their natural good taste whilst working on this project and for finding me funny when I'm drunk. Also big kisses to Dominic and Ben, who don't find me funny when I'm drunk but allowed me to show them up in print anyway.

'I realise that patriotism is not enough.
I must have no hatred or bitterness
towards anyone'

–Edith Cavell

Contents

Thinking Of England

'Can we stop now?' asked Ben, turning blue.

'Give it five more minutes,' I gasped.

'I can't,' he said, letting go of his end of the towel. 'It's taking all the skin off my nipples.'

'It is chafing a bit, isn't it?' I said, reaching for the remote control.

I turned off the video. We were trying the 'Sexercise' workout for an article I was writing. To do the Sexercises properly, you were meant to buy the Sexerciser. Basically, this was a towel with handles at either end to be held by the Sexercising couple and, as it cost twenty pounds, we were making do with Ben's 'Men Of The Florida Keys' bath sheet instead. I did feel the burn at one point but then I realised that I'd dropped my cigarette down the front of my leotard. I know I shouldn't have been smoking while doing the exercises, but the video doctor said that we had to replicate the lovemaking mood as far as possible. For Ben, this should've meant dressing up as Lawrence of Arabia but he couldn't really get his leg up in a burnous.

I'd told Ben that I was undertaking a consumer test and asked him if he would mind playing Cyril Fletcher to my Esther Rantzen. He agreed but had no idea that the Sexercises were merely a warm-up. I had something much bigger in mind.

For a few years I'd made a living writing, mainly on the topic of sex, for a number of women's magazines. I dredged up every experience I'd had in seventeen sexually active years from masturbation to troilism via voyeurism and picking up men in supermarkets. But then I met Dominic, now my husband, and fell in love with him and, more importantly, his tattoos. Pretty soon I realised that I'd covered every notch on my bedpost. Being in a stable monogamous relationship didn't augur well for my career as a sexpert. It looked as if I would end up writing *Family Circle*-type articles on arguments I'd had with Dominic over whose turn it was to load the dishwasher.

So I made a decision. I would go beyond the foot of my own divan and attempt to consumer test the English sexual experience. I was slightly worried that I wouldn't find enough stories out there to keep the dishwasher in Finish for too long as I'd always held the belief that if there was a Eurovision sex contest, Britain would be Portugal – breathless with effort and scoring *deux points*. But in a surge of economically motivated patriotism I felt it was my duty to try and prove otherwise. And to be honest, there were several fantasies I was keen to try out.

It was difficult to know who should act as accomplice

on this investigation. Although Dominic was the obvious choice, I felt that involving my relationship in what was primarily a professional exercise could lead to difficulties. The chief worry would be keeping a proper professional distance from the activities I was looking into. With Ben, who possesses a certain bromide quality, that wouldn't be a problem.

I'd already collaborated with Ben, a fellow journalist, on a number of articles about sex and he was always useful for a quote when I was short of an interviewee, often appearing in the guise of 'Brenda, a twenty-four-year-old midwife who knows a lot about making babies'. Actually, impregnation isn't Ben's strong point as he's gay. (On occasion he does sleep with women but only those who can quote the full filmography of Maria Montez.) Ben's my best friend and there are few secrets between us. Some women always hang around with an ugly friend to make themselves look more attractive. The reason I hang around with Ben is that he makes me look less common.

Perhaps more importantly, Ben has a memory which remains totally unimpaired by years of alcoholic excess. This was essential because I knew that to actually go and do some of the things I planned would mean taking to the drink in a big way to combat nerves. Many's the morning that I've awoken with a shocking hangover and a vague sense of shame, and needed to phone Ben to find out just why I felt so bad. Never once has he been unable to recount in full-colour detail my activities of the night before. Though I curse him for his total recall, it's been useful on occasions when I've needed to retrieve expensive underwear and forgotten where I've left it.

After our Sexercise workout, in what may have been a

post-orgasmic flush or, more likely, the onset of an asthma attack, Ben agreed to help me. Why, was anybody's guess. I think he just liked laughing at people without their clothes on.

From the beginning, we ruled out activities that involved children, animals or cadavers, although by the end of the investigation, I think those last two topics may have been covered. The selection process for our exploits was largely determined by what order invites arrived through my letter-box and the fact that, as is always the case with sex, one thing would lead to another, as there is a big crossover contingent between groups.

Perhaps the single most astonishing thing I discovered while doing this was the incredible amount of bureaucracy involved in becoming a slut. Every group or organisation that I joined sent form after form requiring me to detail at great length the exact nature of my erotic preferences. After a while I realised that I didn't really have any and would just tick yes to all the suggestions provided.

I think all of this bureaucracy is a way of making you feel as if you've achieved something by getting into the club. Many of the groups spoke about their strict vetting procedures, but basically if you're a woman with any one of your three orifices still in action, membership will never be refused. Furthermore, most groups offer discounts to women as an enticement to join. It's something of a buyers' market for 'ladies' (as women on the sex scene are invariably known) as the ratio of men to women in most of these groups is the same as it is in the Osmonds. These discounts are useful because, although a lot of the people on the scene look cheap, you need a full purse to keep up with them.

I fully intended to travel all over England in search of the crack, but my look behind the bedroom nets does have a south-east bias. In the main, this is because most sex events take place in and around London and people travel in from everywhere else. I did try arranging meetings with swingers in Manchester through adverts in *Loot*, but blonde, curvaceous, bi Mandy and her partner, tall, dark, heterosexual Carlos from Whalley Range have yet to answer my call. I don't think the north should feel too snubbed – a lot of what I've seen happening down south isn't too pretty.

In certain cases, I've changed the names of groups and people to protect the guilty. I never wanted to expose anyone. I'm not the kind of person who thinks that a blow job performed by a minor celebrity in a lay-by should be front-page news for a month.

It was hard explaining to some people what I was doing. My mother seemed to take it particularly badly. I tried emphasising the patriotic angle – by showing the world the heat rising off England's Slumberlands, I could restore a nation's pride. I told her that there was really no difference between me and Vera Lynn. She didn't buy it. She took to her bed saying I'd bring shame on the family name. I wasn't too bothered. Mrs Shirley Churchill is a woman who will tell her intimate deodorant preferences to a stranger at the drop of a hat, so the question of shame is relative.

My friends were doubtful that I'd actually find anything worth looking into. In fact, I barely managed to skim the surface. For instance, to name but two examples, I didn't manage to track down the address of The

Corduroy Club (for people who are turned on by, yes, corduroy) and was unable to join The Smoothie Club (for lovers of pubic depilation) as Ben flatly refused to Nair his nether regions. Other people were horrified that I'd even attempt to do something like this. In answer to the question 'Why did I do it?', what can I say? I had to. I was Thinking of England.

Chapter 1

Are You Looking For Action?

Rubber isn't particularly my fetish. Smallbone kitchens are, but I couldn't work out how I could go to the Safer Planet Sex Ball (formerly known as The Sex Maniacs' Ball) dressed as one. The dress code on the ticket gave the theme as rubber, leather, fetish, tribal or space-age. I ruled out space-age knowing I'd never get into my brother's Star Trek pjs. Tribal seemed a bit David Attenborough-y and the last time I'd worn leather trousers Ben said I looked like a Chesterfield. So Dominic (who, despite my reservations, refused to be left out of anything that involved the fetish scene), Ben and I went in search of latex.

I chose a fetishwear shop in north London as my membership of the Safer Planet Sex Club entitled me to a discount there. We stood nervously outside and I instructed the boys to look as if they were *au fait* with fetishism. No sooner had we got through the door than they were fingering the peepholes on a rubber bra and laughing themselves stupid. To distract from their gaucheness, I held a pair of see-through incontinence pants to my waist, announcing loudly something to the effect of, 'They're not as good as the ones that I got from Bart's'. The assistant peered over her facial piercings with an encouraging nod. She could tell that I was a woman who meant business. With nonchalance, I swept an armful of merchandise off the rails and made for the changing room.

What is neglected when talking about rubber fetishism is that the rubber enthusiast has to develop a similar attachment to talcum powder. Getting into rubber without it is a far from smooth ride. At the time I didn't know this. The first rubber dress I tried claimed to be a medium. As I was ignorantly talcum powder-free, I could only wear the dress as a swimming hat. Several medium dresses later, the sounds of twanging elastic drew the attention of the assistant. Peeking her nose ring around the red velvet drapes of the changing room, she helpfully suggested that I try something from their line for the fuller figure and handed me a bottle of Johnson's Baby Talc. Fuller figure? What was she going to give me – something from the Evans' Maîtresse range?

She returned with a size large in red that had only an eraser's worth of extra rubber in it and I disappeared in a mushroom cloud of baby powder. I can't understand why they say rubber fits like a second skin. My dress fitted more like a second spleen. I swished back the curtains for the expected round of applause.

'Five pound of potatoes in a two-pound bag,' said Ben.

I let the fact that I looked like a Big Shopper over-burdened with Marris Pipers ride and bought the dress.

Unable to work out if indeed the peephole bras were for men, we adjourned to a gay sex shop where Dominic and Ben chose their outfits while I deliberated over a leather sling. Finally they picked matching all-in-one wrestler's leotards. Even though Ben is much bigger than Dominic, his vanity wouldn't let him buy anything in a larger size. He has this kind of reverse anorexia problem that when he looks in the mirror he sees somebody half his weight. Therefore his suit was something of a tight fit.

Preparing for the Ball, we hit the Johnson's with a vengeance. Yanking, pinching and scraping, we wormed our way into the outfits. It seemed as soon as one piece of flesh was put under wraps, another would escape in a puff of talc. However, the wonderful thing about latex is that once you do manage to get everything into it, everything stays in place. It's a fabulous way to resculpt your body. You want your bum a couple of inches higher. Hoist it up under rubber and it'll stick. I saw Ben craftily redesigning his love-handles as chest muscles, while Dominic moved some thigh into the groin area to form an attractively full pouch. As a finishing touch, we buffed ourselves up with Starshine, the rubber lover's Mr Sheen.

Judging from fetish magazines I've read, footwear seems to be important for the fetish enthusiast. For men, the look seems to be builder-cum-motorcyclist, while for women, anything goes as long as the heel is above six inches and would look good jammed in someone's mouth. Thinking about it, I may have got that the wrong way round. It's probably the men in the heels, but Ben insisted that his flat feet couldn't support anything more than a sensible court heel. So I plumped for thigh-high patent leather and the boys chose matching biker boots. What was it with the Doublemint Twins? Why did their outfits have to be the same down to the last detail? Dominic suggested that it was a man thing. Even under these strange circumstances, they felt a neurotic need to conform, not to look out of place.

I called a cab and we took one last look at ourselves in the mirror. Dismissing the notion that we looked like a packet of three, I pulled a trench-coat over my dress. I felt that it would be better to travel under wraps so as to not frighten the cab driver. Ben discovered that once he'd pulled on his jeans, he could no longer sit down.

'It's going to blow any minute,' he warned, with the wisdom of Red Adair.

I squeaked my way to the front seat of the cab after laying Ben on his side in the back with Dominic. The smell of rubber was appalling. The cab driver helpfully suggested that it might be his brakes. The Ball was taking place in a warehouse in the Royal Victoria Docks and the driver was curious to know why we wanted to go there so late at night. Noticing a 'Jesus Is Love' sticker on his dashboard, I said nothing. Not that I needed to. As we pulled into the docks, a six-foot 'woman' wearing little more than a corset, crossed in front of the car. I think the driver realised that the bulge in her knickers wasn't a prayer book.

We were vetted at the door by another even taller drag queen, checking we'd met the dress requirements. A bouncer stopped Dominic for looking normal, so I opened my trench-coat, flashed the latex and in we walked. I was delighted to find that the coat-check man was wearing a mac similar to mine. But when he pulled open his lapels, out popped a thrusting set of stick-on bosoms. I couldn't compete.

On our way in, we were given a programme with a map of the building and details of the evening's special attractions. The map showed three interconnecting warehouses. In the first, 'The Stadium', was a disco, a bar and an erotic fairground. The second warehouse, 'The Launch Pad', combined a ritual sacrifice altar, a spacecraft drive-in cinema and the promise of SM Olympics. The third warehouse was called, most enticingly, 'Fuckafuckaland'. Here you could flit from the Tit and Bum Print Room to the Mass Grope Box as your fancy took you.

Among the special events taking place were films at the drive-in which included *Eric Kroll Girdle Photography* and *Virtual Valerie.* This second film was about computer sex, although I had it confused with *Virtually Valerie* which was a film about a pre-operative transsexual called Victor. Over on the main stage the cabaret line-up included the talents of The Thinking Man's Fetish Band and Teena Tormenta, both stalwarts of many a Royal Variety Performance. At one-thirty AM, there were plans for a Cocksucking and Pussy-Eating Competition. Unfortunately, we had arrived too late to see the Dildo Juggling spot. It bugged me that I would never find out if the jugglers used their hands or not.

We chose to start off in The Stadium, eager for a drink and a ride in the erotic fairground. The warehouses were split-level and to get to The Stadium meant navigating a long staircase dotted with some of the most fabulously over- (and under-) dressed people I have ever seen outside of a Stepney wedding. It looked like the finale of a Ziegfield show as designed by Alfred Kinsey. When I first put on the rubber dress I had felt like Betty Page. Next to these people, I looked like Betty Turpin. The thing that surprised me most was the age range of the revellers. Some of them could have been wearing rubber knickers at the Somme.

There was a crowd at the bar. Fighting my way through the tit-clamps and the ciré pouches, I ordered a drink. As I reached into my bag for my purse, my hand grazed against the naked buttocks of a leather-man standing next to me. I knocked back my beer in one. Turning to leave, I bumped into a man, in his sixties, dressed in a blue gingham baby-doll with matching bonnet and a Post-It note pinned to his shoulder saying, 'I am lost. Please return me to the nursery'. I ordered another drink. It was going to be a long night.

In one corner of the warehouse stood an inflatable boxing ring. We sat on the edge of it – that is to say, Dominic and I sat while Ben just leaned against the ropes, still unable to bend – and let the spectacle wash over us. As plain as I now felt in my simple rubber dress, the fact that I had made a nod towards fetishism made it far easier to scrutinise other people. It was a case of you show me yours and I'll show you mine. Had I worn sensible shoes and a pleated skirt, I would have felt like a voyeur. This way I could quite openly stare at the fifty-year-old dominatrix standing next to us administering 'correction' to a woman half her age. I feared for the dominatrix's beehive as it teetered precariously with each thwack of her whip.

Whether it fell or not, I can't say; my attention was

drawn away by two youthful Greek nymphs who floated by in a cloud of golden body paint, the contents of a fruit bowl Sellotaped to their heads. They were quickly followed by a middle-aged woman with exposed and heavily tattooed breasts, her nipples pierced with what seemed to be the kneading attachments from a Magichef. Worried that her husband might be tempted away from her in such fleshy surroundings, she had thoughtfully taken the precaution of putting him on a chain. This chain was attached to a piercing through the head of his exposed penis. Dominic unconsciously clutched his crotch as she passed.

There must have been around two thousand people there. Most of them seemed to fit the remit of the dress code. For instance, on the space-age front, a lot of the men there were dressed like Judy Jetson, and the people from Planet Sex were recognisable by the Space Cadet signs stuck to antennae on their heads. However, the older space fans had to go further back into the past for a vision of what the future would look like and had drawn their inspiration from H.G. Wells – supposing, that is, that the Martians from *The War of the Worlds* wore tinsel wigs.

If I-Spy books had a fetish edition, I'm sure I could have ticked off everything in under an hour. But there were those whose fantasies seemed pretty impenetrable even though they were wearing them on their sleeves. For instance, why was the musketeer look so popular? Actually, I never managed to see more than three at any one time. I wondered if there were groups of Three Sexy Musketeers all over the country who go to these events in the hope of finally meeting up with a D'Artagnan. You can imagine the heartbreak that follows when they spot a lone musketeer and give him the old come hither, only to find out he's another Athos waiting for Porthos and Aramis to come out of the toilets.

Emboldened by drink, I wanted to try one of the rides. Nobody seemed too keen to try bouncy boxing, so the choice was either the Quasar Spaceship or something called 'The Ride of Your Life'. This turned out to be a variation on the bucking bronco machines seen at rodeos. The horse had been replaced with a life-size model of a reclining near naked man. Apparently, you sat in his lap and held on for dear life, which seemed a pretty accurate simulation of the real thing. Alongside the bucking man lay a model of a woman on all fours, ready to step in for the men who thought there was something perverse about bucking with a man. I would have tried it had wearing a latex dress not meant abandoning my knickers.

Not that I necessarily showed any less in the Quasar Spaceship. When I first saw it, I had mistaken it for a bouncy castle. My heart leapt. I could think of nothing more perverse than running about a bouncy castle in a rubber frock. But there was an added attraction with the Spaceship – you were armed with a laser gun and wearing a body harness with targets. The targets were meant to vibrate when you were hit and a woman in the queue behind me was worried that the vibrations might bring on a heart attack. As if running around a bouncy castle in crotchless knickers and a full set of body jewellery wasn't enough to do the trick.

Trying to keep my dress down and my body count up wasn't easy. Ben bounced once, fell over and was unable to get up again. Though he was supposed to be on my team I delighted in shooting the man when he was down. The spirit of the evening had caught me and I felt a surge of Sadeian power. I needed a whip. It was time for Fuckafuckaland.

On my way there, I passed two men who I knew would be the first to feel the kiss of leather on their backs. The first was a suburban bank manager type wearing only bra and panties, which miraculously seemed to fall off any time he went near a kitten with a whip. Clutching a handbag to his privates, he would stick out his bottom and snivel, 'Yes, Mistress. Sorry, Mistress'. I felt the beatings he had received so far were not commensurate with the anger I felt about the interest on my overdraft. Therefore whippee number one.

Number two was a Nazi. Torn between which Nazi he actually wanted to be, he had compromised and come as Adolf and Eva, with the top half tunic, the bottom, fishnets. He was one of a group of three similarly dressed Nazis – sort of Nuremberg's answer to the Beverly Sisters. The head Nazi, or Joy, had taken a shine to my kinky boots and had been pestering me throughout the evening. When I had tried to give him the brush-off, he, along with Babs and Teddy, saluted me with a chorus of *Sieg heils*. I was incensed. Especially because, as they did this, a man dressed as a Hassidic Jew (or possibly the real thing) walked by and shot me a look that said, 'Get you, Leni Riefenstahl'.

The first port of call in Fuckafuckaland was an attraction marked on the outside as a 'Puppet Show'. Ben rushed in, in the hope of seeing Pinky poking Perky or Jeff Tracey involved in a *ménage à trois* with Parker and Lady Penelope. It was actually a peep-show and Ben took his place at the last of the available slits.

'What can you see?' I asked breathlessly.

'Well, she's just pulled her hand out but Sooty's not on the end of it.'

Pushing him out of the way, I looked through the slit to see a middle-aged woman laying on a bed with her legs wide open, masturbating furiously. As I watched agog, I felt a hand on my bum. Thinking it belonged to Dominic, I pressed against it and carried on watching. The show reached its climax and I left with a smile on my face. Dominic was waiting outside complaining that he hadn't been able to get in. It was so dark in there.

I bought a black rubber whip which had a dildo for a handle. The salesman displayed admirable product knowledge by pointing out the depth to which it was okay to insert the dildo (which, as a matter of interest, was several notches above my own Plimsoll line). He also warned me not to hold the whip by the glans or it would tear. I gave it a few practice cracks and named it 'Doris Day' in tribute to the song 'The Deadwood Stage'. I felt empowered.

As I gave Doris a few more swishes, the man in the gingham baby-doll was led past me on the arm of a concerned musketeer. The nursery was a few stalls along from the whip stand. There were around ten adult babies in and around the play-pen. They were dressed in matching outfits though the gingham on the baby girls' dresses was pink. Even with this nod to femininity it was patently obvious that the majority of the baby girls were, in fact, men. One such baby girl was sitting by the pen in a big pram.

I pointed to her and said to Ben, 'I don't understand it.'

'It's obvious,' he replied. 'It's her turn to be pushed.'

'But what's the sexual kick in dressing up like a baby?'

'Maybe they really want to dress up like musketeers but they're masochists.'

Ben refused to see anything wrong with being an adult baby.

'It just looks so odd,' I told him.

'And we look normal?'

Ben was clued up on the subject of sexual infantilism, having seen it on *Oprah*, and lectured me on how I mustn't confuse it with paedophilia, as the two things were at completely different ends of the sexual spectrum.

'Do you think their nappies are full?' asked Dominic, to stop the argument.

It must have been the power of suggestion as I suddenly felt the need to go to the toilet. It was pretty hard to tell if I was in the men's or women's even though everyone in there was wearing a dress. A group of matronly looking women were reapplying their make-up, and their outfits confirmed my suspicions that Evans did do a fetish range. But I had to hand it to them, not every woman looks good in a PVC A-line skirt.

On my way out, I was stopped by a transvestite in a long blonde wig and a biker's cap. I started chatting to him, wrongly assuming that, as he was in the women's toilets in a pair of heels, he was gay. He borrowed my lipstick and touched up his Cupid's bow. Then he turned to me.

'You look saucy,' he said. 'Are you looking for action?'

I fled.

Back on the dance-floor, my whip-hand was beginning to twitch. I watched as one of the old spacemen in the tinsel wigs had his crotch tickled with a riding crop by a woman dressed as a bride. She could have stepped straight from the pages of a Pronuptia catalogue. If the

Pronuptia catalogue also carried a line in strap-on dildoes. I couldn't hold myself back and whipped the spaceman across the back. It nearly gave him a stroke. Calm down, I told myself and then lashed out at another passer-by. I was a woman possessed.

'That was a blind man you just hit,' said Dominic. I felt awful.

'Maybe he was just a man with a fetish about being visually-challenged,' said Ben, to comfort me.

I tracked down the bank manager and laid into him.

'Ooh, thank you, Mistress.'

I gave up after a few swings and gave the whip to Ben. It was no fun when they enjoyed it. Letting go of the whip was a mistake because as soon as I had done so I felt a bullwhip creeping up the back of my thigh. It was Babs the Nazi who frog-marched me on to the dance-floor and made me look like a collaborator. On seeing this, Ben rushed over with Doris Day and rescued me.

'Leave my woman alone,' he said, hitting Babs hard in the tights. The whip (and the drink) had gone to his head.

As further proof of this, when we walked through the drive-in cinema again on our way out, Ben picked me up and threw me on to the bonnet of a car. Unfortunately, the brake wasn't on and the car rolled backwards, disturbing the three naked occupants inside. Apologising profusely through the windscreen, I got down again. There were groups of people standing around each of the cars and Ben felt that it would be a good idea for the three of us to get in one: Dominic and I in the back and Ben in the front acting out his chauffeur fantasy, until I reminded him that he couldn't drive.

Just before we left, I bought a copy of the Planet Sex

Diary which was filled with contact addresses. I wanted to try out everything (bar the adult babies) I'd seen happening around me throughout the evening. From Auto-Eroticism to Zoophilia, I intended to work my way through the book.

Chapter 2

SATURDAY NIGHT BENEATH THE PLASTIC PALM TREES

'Nude ping pong,' said Ben, when I asked which area of sex he thought we should look into first.

Some men grow up with Marmite, with Ben it was *Health and Efficiency*. Many's the hour he had spent throughout his teens poring over pictures of mottled naked flesh taken on windswept British beaches. It wasn't so much the nudity he was interested in as the hairstyles, as *H&E* has the endearing habit of using twenty-years-out-of-date photographs to accompany its articles. Thus, to this day, Ben can still be found in a quiet moment taking a magnifying glass to a picture of nude sun-lovers Maureen and Raymond, sitting on the bonnet of their Morris Minor, parked in the dunes at Holkham Bay, to see if Maureen's hair is up in a lattice-work beehive or merely a classic French pleat.

There were lots of things that Ben wanted to know about naturism. For instance, why, as soon as nudists strip off, do they have the compulsion to play table-tennis? Or why do lady nudists always shave their pubic hair into an oblong wedge? And where could he buy a sun-lounger like the ones featured in the pictures?

I shared Ben's suspicion that naturism wasn't as innocent as its practitioners would have us believe. So, after agreeing with Ben that Tilde, pictured wearing only a belly chain and wielding a ping-pong bat on a verdant hilltop above the Rhine, was indeed sporting a 'Jackie Kennedy', I wrestled the copy of *H&E* out of his hands and found an advert for Rio's, a nudist club in north London, and sent off for a brochure.

When it arrived I read that the club was set in luxurious tropical surroundings, with 'large Finnish sauna, Turkish steamroom, two large Jacuzzis, plunge pool, fully equipped gymnasium, qualified masseuses and satellite TV lounge'. As further inducement to the reluctant 'textile' (nudist lingo for clothes-wearer), Rio's promised complimentary drinks and snacks served at the Tropical Beach Bar by the type of comely tropical beauty who well knew her way around a Bounty Bar.

What does one wear to a nudist club? I made the mistake of picking a lycra top that fastened at the crotch only if somebody else did the press studs. So preparing for my first sortie into sex meant lying on my bed with Ben between my legs, fiddling with my gusset. I couldn't really help as I had a can of beer in both hands owing to a sudden attack of nerves. Anyway, a bit of close-quarter work was good for Ben to re-acquaint himself with the terrain. I remember once asking him to draw what he thought a woman looked like 'down there' and the result looked not unlike the CND logo.

It seemed sensible to start off at a nudist club to get

over the remaining inhibitions, if any, that we had about our bodies. Getting ready to go, we had stood naked in front of a mirror and compared notes. I was bothered by the combined effect that gravity and the Women's Movement had had on my breasts. I didn't want to come home from Rio's having to write the line, 'I stood apprehensively at the end of the diving board, the waves lapping gently at my nipples'. Ben suggested running my fingers repeatedly through my hair, as raising my arms above my head lifted my bosoms a good inch.

He was worried about holding his stomach in all evening. This is a man who's been able to hold his stomach in throughout a five-year relationship so you'll understand that I wasn't duly concerned.

'But it's different naked,' he insisted. 'There's a telltale sign.'

I forced him, under duress, to tell me what it was. There could be no secrets on this journey.

'When I pull my stomach in,' he confessed, 'my balls lift up into my body and my scrotum just hangs there like an empty bum-bag.'

As he demonstrated this phenomenon, Dominic entered the bedroom, shook his head in disgust and walked out again. I'd like to believe that coming upon me in the boudoir nakedly inspecting the disappearing Niagaras of another man had sent a sudden rush of jealousy coursing through his veins, but in truth he was just upset that we'd drunk all the beer.

I was annoyed about being nervous. Going to a nudist club was hardly hands-on stuff. If I couldn't even cope with taking my clothes off in public, how could I possibly manage the challenge I had set myself? It grew worse when we arrived outside the club, which stood bold as brass in the middle of the high street. It called itself a health club; no mention of naturism, no hint of oblong wedge. But there was no getting away from it: it looked like a knocking shop. Fortunately, there was a pub next door.

Several bottles of Pils later, we made our move and found a gang of teenagers heckling the customers as they went in. We went back to the pub. I only knew that I'd reached the point where I was ready to drop 'em when I found myself on stage attached to a Karaoke machine belting out 'Galveston'.

On entering the club, we were handed two bath towels and ushered to separate changing rooms. I was puzzled by this sudden nod to inhibition. Surely the idea was to parade your naked body in front of members of the opposite sex? As I struggled to undo the press studs of my top, with one leg cocked and resting on the door of a locker, I noticed a sign on the wall warning patrons not to ask the qualified masseuses for 'extras', as none was on offer.

When I'd finally got all of my clothes off, I glanced at the bath towel. Was I going to wimp out and wear it? How could I win the respect of the serious naturists out by the plunge pool if I chose to remain textile? I decided to brazen it out. It was my body and it was beautiful. I came out of the changing room, naked, proud and manically running my fingers through my hair.

My heart, that is to say my bosoms, sank at the sight before me. I was standing in the tropical satellite TV lounge. Not only did everyone there have a towel on, all of the women were wearing swimming costumes. I say *all* of the women, there must have been about three others and two of them were obviously on the payroll. I returned to the thankfully women-only changing room and covered my shame. At least with a towel on, I had somewhere to tuck my cigarettes.

I returned to the TV lounge, hoping that nobody would notice the attractive imprints left around my ankles by the elastic in my socks. I spotted Ben, reclining, with towel, on a plastic sun-lounger, feigning marvel at the abundance of plastic bougainvillea that swooped dramatically above his head. He had already made a recce of the place in order to look for fire exits. That week an unlicensed porn cinema in Smithfield had gone up in flames killing eleven people and he wasn't taking any chances. I heard a parrot squawk and memories of a beach in Sri Lanka washed over me. When, seconds later, I heard, note for note, exactly the same parrot squawk, I realised that I was listening to a tape-recording.

I pulled up a sun-lounger next to Ben and sat down, glad to be wearing a towel as the thought of sitting nude on a plastic chair filled me with horror. Things might stick. I asked Ben what he wanted to do, as there didn't seem to be a ping-pong table.

'We could play "Spot the Anus",' he said.

Thinking over his suggestion, I went off to try the bar. I was beginning to warm to the idea of being in a naturist club where nobody took off their clothes. I could easily sit at the Beach Bar in my towel, sip a free Pina Colada from a coconut half-shell and lose myself in the sound of (taped) crashing waves. I could almost smell that bougainvillea.

It was at the Beach Bar that I caught my first sight of naked flesh. Three rather large undressed men were propped up at the counter, their buttocks hanging over the back of their bar stools. I wedged my way in between them, holding my head erect, not wishing to see what was hanging over the front of their bar stools. This was unnecessary as their stomachs acted as aprons shielding their genitalia from view. Should I tell them my secret for sagging breasts, I thought, as I rifled through my hair yet again.

The barmaid was topless and, in my gratitude, I let my towel slip an inch or so.

'A Pina Colada and don't spare the umbrellas,' I intended to say.

'Orange or blackcurrant?' she asked.

Oh, well, a freshly squeezed orange juice in a half-shell and throw in a swizzle stick.

She handed me a plastic beaker half-full with Kia-Ora.

'And snacks?' I ventured.

She pointed to two jars on the bar filled with shortbread fingers, with a look that said, 'My tits are out because they're paid to be.'

Tucking myself in, I took a biscuit back to Ben in the TV lounge where he was craning his neck to watch *The Chief* on a fuzzy black-and-white television hanging above him. He had his towel up around his neck as he was determined that nobody was going to get a good look at his love handles while he was in respite. Around ten other men were sitting watching with him, their towels not so artfully draped, revealing, along with their love handles, the odd sliver of foreskin. The kick in naturism was beyond me.

'Why do you think they want to come here and sit on a plastic chair, drink squash and watch black-and-white telly?' I asked Ben.

'Perhaps all their chairs are Dralon at home,' he replied.

Much to everybody's consternation the screen suddenly went blank. Though there was some novelty value to watching a spot of nude TV repair, we decided to try one of the Jacuzzis. They were mounted on plinths and to get in, I had to duck to avoid the suspended ceilings.

Ben and I had the Jacuzzi to ourselves for about five minutes and then we were joined by the three men who had been at the bar. It was a tight squeeze getting us all in. As I shifted to put some room between me and an encroaching thigh, I sat directly on a hot-water jet, lost my grip on the side and turned upside down with my legs sticking out of the water. God knows what I pulled on to right myself but Ben was hysterical.

'I spotted one,' he said.

The three men looked pleased that they'd spotted one too.

Not that they were unhappy looking at my breasts.

'Look at them,' whispered Ben. 'You've got three hungry mouths to feed there.'

They were staring rather a lot. One of them was democratic enough to be sitting in a position where his penis was just breaking the surface of the water so I could stare back if I chose. I chose not to. Ben stood up to get out first so that the men would get out of the way for me. As he pulled himself out, he slipped on a step and fell, scraping his arm down the Artexed wall and ended up on all fours outside of the Jacuzzi.

'Spotted one too,' I said, stepping over him and going into the steamroom.

Eight naked panting men and me. When I first went into the steamroom I was in there panting by myself. Then Ben joined me, followed soon after by the three men from the Jacuzzi and four from the TV lounge which meant seven eyes to a nipple.

Swinging my legs nervously back and forth, I turned to the man sitting next to me and asked, with blinding originality, 'Do you come here often?'

He said he did as he liked the relaxing and healthy atmosphere. By 'healthy' I took it that he meant the ten position home gym from Argos which stood in a room at the back. He seemed reticent on why he was a 'naturist' but I assumed it was to catch the odd flash of muff like every other man in the steamroom.

'Does anything else happen here?' I asked, noticing that the man sitting opposite me had a penis of such a length he should have really worn a verruca sock on the end of it.

He claimed that nothing did, but if I wanted a more 'liberal' atmosphere there was a club in Kent called Eureka that I could try. Noticing that the heat was stirring up the alcohol in me, I decided it was time to go.

On my way back through the TV lounge, I dropped my cigarettes and as I bent over to pick them up my towel fell off. Ben was standing behind me.

'Do I get any points for seeing the same one twice?' he asked.

Textile again, we left and hailed a cab.

'Did you find it exciting?' I asked.

'No I did not,' said Ben. 'There wasn't a single woman there who knew how to backcomb.'

Chapter 3

THE SMELL
OF
BURNING RUBBER

Having enjoyed the Safer Planet Sex Ball, we were quite keen to try out more of the fetish scene. The first club we joined was Submission. Ben said that if we were going to do this on a regular basis then he would have to have a new outfit, as he wasn't sure if his wrestling suit could stand the strain.

Ben had read an article about the Fetish Market that was held every second Sunday of the month in west London. Eager to outdo me and Dominic at Submission, he sneaked off one Sunday morning to the address given, accompanied by his friend who wanted her navel pierced. Afterwards he phoned to confess all.

'So did Liz have her belly button done?' I asked, mildly annoyed that he'd gone off without me.

'No.'

'Why not?'

'Because when we got there, all we found at that address was a branch of Citibank.'

My clued-up research assistant hadn't been able to glean from the address that it was, in fact, just a box number. I wrote off to find out the real address and a couple of weeks later we drove to a club in Putney. Anticipation was running high but to be truthful the most exciting part of the afternoon was sitting in the Fetish Market café eating steak and kidney pie.

There were around fifteen stalls in the market and judging from the clientele we could have been at a boot fair in aid of the local branch of the Conservative Party. Most of the people there were dressed in their non-fetish Sunday best and a lot of the women looked as if they were probably just as keen whipping up something for the WI as they were flagellating their husbands.

It didn't take long to realise that in the world of fetishism there are only so many variations on a theme. Most items can be fitted into two categories. There are those items which in some way prohibit normal bodily functions. And there are the weapons. On sale in the former category were such items as gags, cock-rings, harnesses, handcuffs (one set on sale were, the vendor proudly informed me, formerly used by Eastern Bloc police), shoes which were designed to be of such a height they would break the wearer's ankles, and lace tutus with waist-deforming corsets. In the latter category, there was a large array of whips, swords and canes.

The one stall that did catch my eye sold buggies for SM gymkhanas. The slave, or in this case, pony, was attached to the buggy with wrist restraints and a bridle. The maker was keen to point out that the buggy was completely portable and could be taken apart to fit in the boot of my car. Sensing my interest, he tied a petite woman in frilly underwear to the cart's handles and instructed her to tow his eighteen-stone frame around the club for a bit of dressage. The resultant spectacle brought to mind a Shetland pony pulling a brewer's dray. At £225 the cart was a little bit too expensive for an impulse buy but I filed away the idea for future reference. If Ben didn't toe the line in future, he could end up towing me.

The anaemic atmosphere at the Fetish Market wasn't really conducive to indulging in one's sexual fantasies and so, aside from picking up a flyer for a fetish party to be held on a pleasure cruiser, we came away empty-handed.

A few days later, I was sitting in my kitchen, in the rubber dress, ready to go to Submission.

'I've got a surprise for you,' shouted Dominic from the top of the stairs. 'Close your eyes. You're not going to believe how sexy this looks.'

Determined to find something new, Dominic and Ben had spent the afternoon shopping. Dominic had felt that it was time to indulge in his own particular sexual fantasy. I closed my eyes.

'You can look now,' he said in a strangely muffled voice. 'Don't you think this looks hot?'

I opened my eyes to see Dominic standing in front of me wearing a pair of leather trousers and naked from the waist up. His face was covered by a US Marine gas mask complete with extendible breathing tube. He had spent over £40 to look like an anteater. It was a good five minutes before I could stop laughing long enough to answer his question. In fact, the laughter was enough of an answer in itself. He looked crestfallen and his breathing tube seemed to droop ever so slightly.

Ben followed on behind him and he hadn't fared much better. He had run the wrestling outfit through a bowl of water to check for leaks and was happy to wear it again.

'But,' he said, delving into his shopping bag, 'the art of wearing the same outfit twice, is the clever use of accessories.'

With this, he produced a pair of thick armpit-length rubber gloves and put them on.

'What do you think?'

'You've an air of James Herriot about you,' I replied, resuming my hysterics.

They had also bought me a pair of gloves, but after wearing them for five minutes I began to lose all sensation in my fingers. If I was going to wear them I would have to carry the whip in my teeth.

Like all fetish clubs, Submission had a strict dress code. On arriving at the club, with our normal clothes covering up our outfits, we found that this code was implemented by the same bouncer who had stopped Dominic at the Ball for being too ordinary. Dominic was stopped again and warned about the 'Tranny Bag'.

For those people who wanted to go into the club and had left their gas mask at the dry cleaners, the 'Tranny Bag' provided the answer. In front of us in the queue, two Japanese businessmen in suits were playing lucky dip. One pulled out a simple but sexy red teddy and the other something that looked like a bin-liner. With a yen for ritual humiliation being built into the Japanese psyche, the two took to their new outfits immediately.

I recognised a lot of the faces at Submission from the Ball. In fact, the first person I spotted on my way in was the transvestite who had accosted me in the toilets. Again he was loitering with intent by the powder rooms. Ben was sure that he had seen his Aunt Josie swish past, although the next day when he phoned his mother to check, she assured him that Josie was too cheap to have pierced nipples so unless they were clip-ons it wasn't her. 'Josie' had given her piercings an airing by shoving the whole cup of her Dorothy Perkins bra underneath her breasts thus cleverly combining her dual needs for exhibitionism and uplift.

In the main, the crowd was younger and more trendy than the Planet people, though a few third-agers had gamely forsaken their Sanatogen and slippers to be there. There was something very celebratory about the club. I had mistakenly assumed that the fetish scene would be very dark and threatening. I was quite sure that the emphasis would be on pain and humiliation, that there would be a fascistic attitude towards bodies. At Submission all seemed welcome. Whether overweight, heavily pregnant, old or disabled in some way, the body could be recognised as erotic. Who knows, somebody may have even found something to celebrate about my cellulite. Maybe not.

As the emphasis seemed to be more on the outfit than the body, it must be said that some people hadn't quite got the look off pat. For instance, there was a very good-looking man with a fabulous body wearing only a leather G-string – and a pair of nylon socks and beige loafers. In fact, there were quite a few men similarly attired, so maybe artificial fibres and slip-on footwear have their own special place on the fetish scene. Another discon-certing sight was a man in a ciré see-through body suit with the most unattractive pair of blue Y-fronts showing through. He had obviously bared as much as he dared but I'm sure showing his bedroom furniture would have been less aesthetically offensive.

Actually, that's probably not true. We were sitting in an alcove taking a breather when a man clad in a pair of leather chaps and a studded codpiece came past attending to a bout of Jock itch. As he scratched on the codpiece, a testicle escaped and screamed for mercy, inches from my face. It wasn't a good look. Meanwhile, Ben was having problems with his gloves. He was completely unable to move his hands in them. Throughout the evening, I had to slot cigarettes in between his immobile fingers and then watch fearfully as he tried to avoid setting himself alight. It would be like a fire in a Michelin factory: he could burn for days.

Dominic too was finding it difficult to smoke. Stubbornly refusing to remove his gas mask, he had me administering blowbacks through the breathing tube. As I exhaled the visor would fog up and wisps of smoke escape from around the mask's edges. It was difficult to know if he was enjoying it in there. He finally admitted defeat after trying to drink lager in a similar fashion. He managed the first couple of chugs okay. But then he choked and, looking like an elephant with *la grippe*, blew half a pint of liquid back out of the tube.

Fetish wear just isn't practical. If it was, my mother would wear it to the supermarket instead of a velour leisure suit. I saw a man with a mask that completely covered his head and where his mouth should have been there was a large zipped-up zip. Unfortunately, the manufacturer had cut the eye slits a good inch lower than anatomically feasible. Hence, the man could see absolutely nothing. Which is probably how he came to lose his friends, George and Bungle. Towards the end of the evening I watched a woman in full body harness slow-grinding with her partner, blissfully unaware that her pudenda had blown its cover.

That's as far as any overt display of sexuality went that evening. Going for a walk around the club, I found an upstairs area divided from the rest of the room by a sheet hanging from the ceiling. I thought that I could smell sex. Ducking under the sheet I saw a fifth generation copy of a porn tape fuzzily panting away on a TV screen. On screen, Blondie was working her tush off trying to accommodate a flock of lobster-coloured penises. Off screen, there were around thirty people watching and not a flicker of interest from any of them. I've seen more tumescence in a Comfort commercial.

Letting the curtain fall on this orgy, I braved the toilets. The sound of twanging latex ricocheted from each of the cubicles. Waiting my turn, I felt a hand on my shoulder.

'Haven't I met you somewhere before?' said the saucy tranny, for it was he.

I explained that we had indeed met.

'You look saucy. Are you looking for action?'

At that point a cubicle door opened and, relieved, I locked myself in and added my own contribution to the sound of the rubber band. However, the tranny was persistent and waiting for me when I came out.

'My name's Mark. Do you know what you're getting into here?'

'What do you mean?'

'Well, you know, Sub/Dom. What are you?'

'What are you?' I asked, avoiding the question.

'Both. Whatever you want.'

I was saved from having to answer by a bouncer bursting into the toilets. 'There are men in here and it's not allowed,' he barked.

How could he tell?

Back on the dance-floor, the eyeless Zippy was still bumping into walls and Ben and Dominic were dancing around my clutchbag. I got talking to a very tactile man named Tony. Tony was a committed fetishist and devoted father, and at that point in the evening completely under the influence of Ecstasy. I listened to a twenty-minute monologue on how adorable and perfect his baby was and how nature was a wonderful thing. His rhapsody was only stopped by the arrival of his wife who snatched him away to prevent him experiencing any more of nature with me.

On leaving the club, I was stopped again by Saucy Mark. Ben was in charge of Doris Day that evening and after a quick flick of the whip, Saucy Mark took his attentions elsewhere and we left. The evening had been a trifle dull. Though wearing the clothes made me feel sexy, there was no follow through. You can't just buy into a fantasy. Putting on a latex dress no more made me a fetishist than putting on a blue hat would make me the Queen Mum. Maybe this sex thing was more difficult than I thought.

Chapter 4

ALL NIPPLES
AND
NET CURTAINS

'Your Uncle Frank and Auntie Bernice are swingers.'

I was shocked. I had phoned my mother to give her a run down on my night in a rubber dress and had happened to mention that I was planning to join a swingers' club. How did she know that Frank and Bernie, a very respectable couple who live in a mobile home park just outside London, were swingers?

'They have parties where the men throw their caravan keys into the ring.'

'What for?' I asked, knowing full well what for but I wanted to hear her say it. Mrs Shirley Churchill isn't a natural when it comes to matters of the groin. Thinking of England? This is a woman who lies back and thinks of Brentford Nylons.

'They swap,' she said knowledgeably.

'Swap what?'

'You know, wives. But I think Frank'd be better off

swapping Bernie for a new Calor gas heater. It's freezing in that caravan.'

See what I mean? Actually, I think my mother's revelation embodies the true spirit of swinging in Britain. I'd always harboured the suspicion that swinging was a provincial pastime, all nipples and net curtains. And now, having had my knees burnt by the shag pile of that particular scene, I know that my suspicions were spot-on.

I found the address of the Party Susan Club in the back of *Loot* (next to an advert for transvestite makeovers which made me think instantly of a new research area for Ben) and sent away for a brochure. Of course, it's not called the Party Susan Club but one of the club rules states, 'Members shall not annoy or bring discredit to the club or its members and shall be discreet about all matters . . .' After all, they still have my address.

The club was started in 1988 after the directors, Adam and Moira, had sampled the British swinging scene and found it wanting. It, according to the brochure, immediately became *the* couples club to join. The brochure went on, 'What makes it work is the proven combination of contact listings, magazines, newsletters and social events *plus* the genuine, active, enthusiastic membership. They're discreet. They're selective. They're very special, fun-loving people'. I can now tell you they are also the kind of people who can spot the difference between 'Muffin' and 'Misty Buff' on a paint chart at fifty paces.

I know that now, but when I was filling in my application to join, I indulged in a fantasy where this particular area of bedroom Britain would be the one to really set me on fire. I imagined semis in Surbiton filled to their add-on porches with glamorous and groaning cost analysts licking honey off the thighs of their Rotary wives. So I wanted to present myself on the form as the kind of woman equally at home with leaded lights or troilism.

Of course, I needed a partner. I asked Ben as I felt resisting the temptations of the flesh and maintaining a professional detachment would be a lot harder if Dominic accompanied me to an orgy. Ben had strong reservations about joining the swinging scene because he was convinced that all the men would be wearing white slip-on shoes but agreed to come as long as Dominic did the TV make-over. Ben argued that he was already fully in touch with his inner woman and an unreconstructed heterosexual man like Dominic could benefit from an afternoon spent in a Cross-Your-Heart bra. Plus he felt that, at last, he had familiarised himself with the territory and could find his way round a vulva should the need arise.

He wasn't too happy when, filling in the application form, I gave his occupation as painter and decorator and mine as secretary. He thought that it sounded too down-market and that we'd only be matched up to swap with couples of a similar ilk. I had to keep reminding him that we weren't a couple and we were definitely not going to swap. If anybody was to ask, he was to tell them we were strictly voyeurs.

As part of my introduction to the Party Susan Club, I got to place an ad in their *Contact Masterlist*. After much deliberation I came up with the following: 'He, twenty-eight, submissive; she, thirty-four, dominant, both bisexual. We are a fun-loving, attractive couple who would like to swap horny letters with photos if possible and meet like-minded couples and singles who are truly bisexual'. We felt that there was something for everyone in that list. I picked 'dominant' as it would allow me to hit anybody who came on too strong and the 'horny letters with photos' would give us some indication of what we were letting ourselves in for before going to any parties. With hindsight, I would have made one important change. Never give any indication that you are open to suggestions from single men – there is normally a good reason why they're single. Wisely, I now feel, I did say no to hosting parties with the club's support. Flushed with the feeling that my description fitted us to a tee I sent off our £40 six-month membership fee and waited for the invites to parties, trips and discos (and let's not forget the horny letters) to come flooding in.

A few days later, I received a letter from the club containing the Masterlist and a run down of the activities planned for the coming months. I scoured the contact ads to find ours and was embarrassed to find that it was by far the most explicit. Some of the others were so vague they could have been advertising for a fourth hand at bridge. I was perturbed by so many people describing themselves as 'clean' as it had the effect of suggesting exactly the opposite. Even if you are scrupulous about scrubbing your underneath, picking 'clean' as one of your most distinguishing attributes speaks volumes about your lack of others.

Of course, all of the men advertising were Well Endowed (WE) or indeed VWE. It would be a brave man indeed who admitted to being NVWE amongst these stallions. Likewise, a lot of people mentioned that they had a GSOH. I spent ages plumbing my sexual lexicon looking for words to fit that acronym until Ben pointed out that it meant Good Sense of Humour. These things are all relative of course and I was pretty positive that the majority of men on offer had dicks like shoelaces and ANSOHAA (Absolutely No Sense Of Humour At All).

One advert did get me going, though. It read, 'Very attractive couple with luxury lifestyle seek truly bisexual female who, once relationships have formed, would like to move into their large country house and share a life of worldwide travel, horses, socialising and blissful sexuality . . .' I could quite easily put out for a stately home and regular trips to the Easter Islands. But I decided against replying. There was something very suspicious about mentioning horses and blissful sexuality in the same sentence.

If I were to apply for the luxury lifestyle, I would make sure that I followed the helpful hints on replying to other swingers thoughtfully provided by the club. When the replies started pouring in, I began to wonder if maybe not everybody had read them thoroughly enough:

Hint 1. Look for shared interests as indicated in each personal advertisement. Just where in our advert did we indicate that we would be interested in watching 'toilet-training videos' with a nightwatchman from Brighton?

2. Don't be too put off by geography. That special meet could be worth the journey! Dear Harry from Hants. It wasn't the geography that put me off: I wouldn't touch your beautifully photographed 'quite WE cock' if it was only a Hoppa away.

3. Do use quality writing paper. Try typing if your handwriting is not that good. Judging from some of the scrawl we received, not using a typewriter does leave a hand free for masturbation.

4. Enclosing a good photo helps. Avoid passport-type photos, they're seldom flattering. The trouble with not sending passport-type photos is that the ordinary sort can show off too much of your soft furnishings. In seventeen sexually active years, I've never once experienced an orgasm on a candlewick bedspread and I'm not about to start now.

5. Do not send full-frontal pics with your first letter. Rita from Wolverhampton craftily got around this rule by only sending photocopies of full frontal pics. Though, from the murky quality of the reproductions, I wasn't actually sure if I was looking at a fully frontal Rita. It could just as easily have been some snaps of the Chunnel.

6. An SAE will help ensure a quick reply. Was that a Stamped Addressed Envelope or a Simply Awesome endowment?

7. Write fully about yourselves and how you think you match the desires of the advertisers. Does a letter that says little more than, and I quote, 'Please write back to me as nobody else ever does', suggest someone who could fully match your desires?

8. REMEMBER – you will be judged by the first impression your letter makes. The above plea came from a man called, I kid you not, 'Mr Ricketts'. What first impression would a Mr Ricketts make on you?

One of the most important pieces of advice the guide gave was, 'Avoid brown envelopes. We all know it's cheaper but it makes you look cheap too!' So now we know. Sending off letters detailing your desire to have every orifice plugged by huskies along with Polaroids showing a great deal of proctological exposition won't make you look cheap unless you send them in a brown envelope. It was hard to know what to do with these letters, bearing in mind that Club Rule 5 states, 'Members will *always* respond to letters received. Offenders are certain to lose their membership'. If any of you reading this are still waiting for me to get back to you then can I take this opportunity just to say thank you. And no thanks.

Shortly after the first batch of letters came an invite to a swingers buffet to be held in a Kensington hotel. I RSVPed that I'd be delighted to attend their 'Finger Food and Fondle' affair and could they please send me their information pack on 'What Happens At A Couples Get Together Evening'?

This hadn't arrived by the day of the party but I took things in my stride. Adam and Moira were probably far too busy piping Philadelphia into vol-au-vent cases to attend to their correspondence. Ben, on the other hand, was feeling the strain. After seeing Rita and Harry airing their privates in public, he was beginning to wish that he'd plumped for the falsies. He had spent the day trying to procure Valium and when that had failed he settled for a six-pack and his most passion-killer knickers. He felt sure that nobody would be aroused by the sight of him in his Mickey Mouse drawers and I can only say he was right.

I, on the other hand, was going for sexy. Adam had written on the invite that it was fine for the ladies to dress sexily as long as they didn't frighten the bellhops on the way in. As I sat on my bed doing up my suspenders, Ben walked into the room and threw the Chunnel pictures at me. I took a long hard look at Rita's aperture and swapped the stockings for something with a reinforced gusset.

We arrived at the hotel nearly an hour late after repeatedly stopping the cab for Ben to go for a wee. At the reception desk, I felt myself redden as I asked for Adam Brown's suite. I was sure the receptionist thought I was a slut and I wanted to flash him my gusset to prove that I wasn't. The room was on the third floor. In the lift, I quizzed Ben on our story.

'How long have we been together?'

'Five years.'

'Married?'

'No, but maybe a summer wedding.'

'Any children?'

'One daughter, Betty, aged two.'

'Why are we late?'

'The baby-sitter couldn't make it and a friend stepped in. So we might have to leave early.'

'What do we say to people who want sex?'

'That your yeast infection has Chambourcy licked.'

'And how much do you charge to rag-roll a dining-room?'

I knocked on the door of Suite 209. The door flew open and a bald man in his late fifties in cream slacks and white shoes, slapped a name tag on my left breast. I could see I would be spending all evening fending off enquiries as to what the other one was called. I guessed from his lack of name tag that this must be Adam. He

ushered us into the bedroom of the suite and introduced us to a small, elegant woman in her early sixties
whose left breast was named Kath.

'Hello,' she said, holding out her hand. 'Have you
ever been to a Harvester's before?'

We both looked blank.

'It's your first time, isn't it?'

'We haven't got a baby-sitter,' burbled Ben.

Kath looked blank.

Sensing that we had reached an impasse, Kath showed
us into the suite's living-room, reached by passing
through the bedroom. The presence of two double beds
unnerved Ben so much he grabbed hold of my waist from
behind and was stuck to my back like a limpet. As we
Flanagan-and-Allened our way into the living-room, I kept
my head bowed just in case the other guests had already
started. I needed a drink before I could play nude Twister.

Adam and Moira hadn't pushed the boat out laying
on a spread. There were three boxes of sweet vinegar, a
bottle of Blue Nun and two plates of artfully arranged
Twiglets. Knocking back a glass of wine, I asked Kath,
'What Happens At A Couples Get Together Evening?'

'Didn't you get your information sheet?'

'No.'

'Well, nothing happens usually.'

I felt Ben slightly loosen his grip on my stomach.

'Not for a few hours anyway. People take a long time
to get going.'

Ben's fingers jabbed my intestines.

Loosened by the drink, I felt able at last to look around
the room. There were around fifteen other couples present, mostly in their early thirties and all thankfully

clothed, not a Chunnel in sight. They all seemed fairly respectable. Surely there couldn't be a toilet trainee amongst them? The snatches of conversation I heard centred on jobs and cars. On the surface it could have been your average office party. The normality of it did little to calm Ben's nerves and, still holding on to me, he frog marched me into the bathroom, unwilling to be left alone for even a second to relieve his bladder.

When we came out, somebody had hit the dimmer switch and most of the swingers were smooching to soft rock classics. We stood against the wall and watched. Next to us, a woman called Sue was smooching with her partner, Beppe. At first, I suspected Sue was a transvestite but Ben, who has an amazing eye for hairpieces, assured me that if she was, she would be wearing a better wig. Wiggy, as we cleverly dubbed her, was wearing Marje Proops glasses which assured her a clearer view of Beppe, who, a foot smaller, was nestling somewhere in her cleavage. I looked at Ben.

'Not if my life depended on it,' he said.

I scoured the room looking for possible talent as Eric Clapton launched into 'Wonderful Tonight'. Eric obviously hadn't seen the trouser on offer at the Party Susan Club. Castro-clone moustaches and Burton 'fun' shirts seemed to be the order of the day; there was a hint of the chip shop about all of them. There were also more white shoes on show than in *Emergency Ward Ten*. Their ladies were mostly bottle blondes (the preferred shade L'Oreal's 'Myra', I think) approximating 'sexy' in leatherette skirts and plunging necklines. One brunette stood out from the crowd. This was because she was of a height that made Beppe look like Meadowlark Lemon. I found her a reliable gauge as to the mood of the crowd:

slowly, throughout the evening, her clothes seemed to melt away.

As snotty as I was being about the swingers, there was no getting away from the fact that they weren't the slightest bit interested in me. I felt snubbed. I dragged Ben on to the dance-floor and we bumped and ground like pros. Not a dickie bird. Perhaps these people knew that we hadn't put 'clean' in our advert. As we swung around the room, I licked my lips in a lascivious manner like they do in porn films. Nothing. I shook my Kitty sticker at a passing moustache. Still nothing. I felt I had toilet trainee written all over my face.

The music came to a stop. Adam was in charge of the DJ-ing and he couldn't find his Beverley Craven tape in the dark. A new couple had come into the room. They were first timers. I could tell that from their Underneath the Arches body posture. Stopping only to drain off the last of the vinegar, I went over and introduced myself, that is to say I pointed to my breast and smiled. Ben assumed his position jammed up against my back.

I was right. It was Paula and Steve's first time. They had walked around the block several times before plucking up the courage to come in. Paula was a secretary and Steve was a cab driver. Like us they had seen the advert in *Loot*. I asked them why they had come.

'Well,' said Steve, 'we've been together six months now and we thought this might make a change.'

Six months? Six months into an affair, I'm still doing it with the lights off. God knows what Steve had up his sleeve for the seven-year itch. Trying not to betray my surprise I ploughed on with the questions. It was hard to concentrate when I knew that they were thinking, 'This woman wants to shag us'.

'Do you go both ways?' I asked Paul.

'Definitely not,' he said, eyeing Ben suspiciously.

'Do you think swinging is about desiring another person, or will any old body do? Is it just about orifices?'

Paula looked confused and then piped up with, 'You should be a journalist, all those questions you ask.'

My mouth fell open but Ben stepped in with, 'She used to be in telephone sales. She never stops when we're at home'.

His 'let's indulge wifey' tone was too convincing and I elbowed him in the stomach.

'Our baby-sitter didn't turn up,' he gasped.

The conversation seemed to dry up. They had given us the once over and Steve was obviously terrified by the idea that Ben wanted to penetrate him. Fortunately, the silence was broken by Adam joining us to ask how we were enjoying the party.

'Who's Victor Meldrew?' Paula whispered, pointing to Adam.

I introduced Adam to the débutants.

Struggling for something to say I came up with, 'And where's the lovely Moira this evening?'

He choked back a Twiglet and said, 'She left me six weeks ago. She's gone to the States and she's not coming back. But all the hurt and the anger have gone now'.

My, emotions fly fast on the swinging scene. Six weeks to get over a five-year relationship? Paula and Steve nodded sympathetically at Adam. It was the kind of timescale they were working to.

'I'm ready for a new relationship,' affirmed Adam. He looked at me with a glint in his eye. 'Do you want to dance?'

'The ladee in reeeed is dancin' with meee.'

Round and round the room I twirled with Adam's thigh twanging my gusset. I looked over his shoulder imploringly at Ben but he was still involved in a stand off with Steve.

'Laadee in reeeed . . .' sang Adam into my ear.

'Have you slept with Kath?' I asked, trying to prise his fingers off my buttocks.

'Of course,' he said, grabbing them tighter. 'Ladee in reeeed . . .'

'I think this is a Gentleman's Excuse Me,' said Ben, finally coming to my rescue. He led me away and I toasted his manliness with another glass of Blue Nun.

By now, I was decidedly squiffy. There still didn't seem to be any sex going on but I knew the crowd was warming up as the petite brunette barometer was down to her stockings and suspenders. I say stockings but I doubt if her little legs could accommodate much more than a pop sock. The anticipation was getting unbearable. Why didn't somebody just go ahead and do it? Well somebody did go ahead and do it. Me. To the complete horror of Paula and Steve, I took my breasts out. This is a real problem I have. Something happens to me at parties. As soon as things seem to be getting dull, out come my bosoms. I think my breasts have a Pavlovian relationship to boredom.

It was like somebody had fired a starting pistol. Ben reacted with speed in returning my breasts to their rightful place but Paula and Steve shot out on to the hotel balcony to hide. Wiggy also saw my bosoms as a sign and had removed her knickers. She was sitting on the settee with one leg hooked over Kath whilst some moustache, not Beppe, got her glasses steamed up with some digital loveplay. I felt the Liebfraumilch churn inside me.

I only just made it to the bathroom in time. Heaving violently over the bowl, I noticed that Ben was pissing into the sink. So did Paula and Steve who came in behind us, obviously thinking the bathroom was a better place to lock themselves away. They didn't stay. Adjusting his dress, Ben pleaded with me to go home. Ten more minutes, I promised him and he went off to find our coats. Sitting on the toilet, collecting my thoughts, I was joined by a man with two glasses and the last of the wine. I think he felt that as I was drunk and already had my underwear around my ankles, one more glass should do the trick. Fortunately, Ben called me from the hallway and I escaped.

'Look at that,' he said, pointing into the bedroom.

On one of the beds, I could see Wiggy's bottom bouncing up and down atop the prone body of the fingering moustache. Beppe was not perturbed as he was active on the other bed servicing a woman from behind. As she was face down I couldn't see her name tag. Beppe was delighted to perform for a crowd and slowed down his strokes, allowing us to view his manhood more clearly. He was clearly expecting applause. Or a standing ovation. I lurched back into the living-room and was cornered by Adam. He led me to the couch where I passed out, face down in his lap.

Ben shook me awake. Apparently, I was there for about three quarters of an hour. Thankfully, I didn't seem to have a particularly nasty taste in my mouth. Aside from the sick. Ben insisted that we leave. He assured me afterwards that he had spent those forty-five minutes talking to a New Zealand woman about stippling a mantelpiece, but I'll never know for sure. We had to go back into the bedroom again to get our coats and amazingly, Wiggy was still bouncing away, her hair-piece having slipped a good inch. I had an overwhelming urge to smack her bum. So I did. Repeatedly. She responded by bouncing faster. Ben threw my mac at me in disgust and marched me out of the hotel.

Chapter 5

PURE TORTURE

With the outlay on clothing and accoutrements, and the various membership fees that I'd paid, embracing the fetish scene was beginning to feel like an expensive mistake. The initial burst of feeling sexy and uninhibited in latex had subsided; quite frankly, worming my way into the dress again was something of a chore. In the hope of finding something new to revive my jaded palate, I had been with Ben and Dominic to a fetish-wear shop called Regulation. I tried on several dresses, each more bizarre than the last. Each outfit brought gales of laughter from the boys. The last dress I tried on was made from black PVC and had metal spikes sticking out from the bosoms.

'A fabulous way to serve nibbles at parties,' observed Ben. 'Cheese and pineapple on one, and sausages on the other.'

And so the red dress made another appearance on

the fetish scene. Torture Garden promised a multi-environment four-level venue featuring, amongst other things, piercing stalls, brain machines, fetters suspension and a performance by Leigh Bowery. As Mr Bowery had, at a previous show, given himself an enema just prior to going on stage and then evacuated his bowels over the assembled audience of ladies and gentleman of the Press, we were less than disappointed to find, on arrival at the club, that his performance had been cancelled due to illness.

I had a feeling of *déjà vu* about Torture Garden. Ben was stopped on the way in by the same bouncer who had stopped Dominic at the Ball and Submission. Again, the bouncer's concern was that Ben looked 'too ordinary'. I'd never heard anybody say that about Ben before and I'm sure the security man who checked Ben's bag and pulled out Doris with a look of horror was prepared to vouch for Ben's oddness.

And, of course, the first person I saw inside was my saucy friend, TV Mark. It was gratifying to find that even such a hardened fetishist as he felt comfortable turning up to a club for the third time in the same outfit. The nylon socks and loafers brigade were also out in force again. One man had given this classic look a new twist by replacing the old codpiece with a pair of artificial-fibre panties held up by a studded leather belt.

Submission had been bright and breezy and had lulled me into a false sense of security about the fetish scene. The mood at Torture Garden was noticeably darker with a stronger emphasis on pain. Visuals of the tattooed and the tormented were being projected on to screens around the club and the sounds of Gregorian chants wafted down from the levels above us. Beforehand, I had half persuaded Ben to have his nipple pierced at the club for documentary purposes; once there, he refused point blank to let anyone near his (in his words) 'raspberries'. I think his reluctance may have had something to do with the videos that were playing on the monitors around the club.

These videos captured the art of body piercing in gorgeous Technicolor close-up. One after the other, the subjects on camera stripped to show a fine assortment of charm bracelets hanging from their nether regions. One woman opened her legs to reveal what I can only describe as a twattoo. Her pubis, which, judging from the complete absence of hair, had probably been subjected to electrolysis, was entirely covered in a tattoo of flames that emanated from her vagina and snaked their way down to lick around her anus. Her labia were of note too, due to the fact that they were completely absent. She was in the process of having a dainty sleeper inserted through her clitoris. Presumably, this would provide her future lovers with a rough guide of where they should be aiming.

The men in the videos were scarcely less inventive. I could foresee problems getting through airport security for the lot of them. One man seemed to have a whole curtain-rail's worth of rings going through his testicles, topped only by the number he had piercing the shaft of his penis. Another had a kind of metal catheter inserted into his dick, carefully locked into place by a bolt which perforated the penis head. The ball stretchers dumbfounded me the most. There were clips of several men who had stretched their balls with metal rings until their scrotums had reached lengths of nine or ten inches.

When you were a child did you ever play games with a tennis ball in a stocking? I think these men may have.

Tearing myself away from the images on film, I looked at the people watching them. Quite a few had facial piercings. How many of them had tennis balls in stockings too? I'd had enough of the videos. I could have stayed at home and watched *Casualty* if I'd wanted to see that kind of thing. We walked up to Level 3, the fetish body-art market, with me firmly clutching on to Doris for protection. In the market, enthusiastic devotees were haggling over the price of second-hand fetishwear. Buying a used car is one thing but second-hand fetishwear? Even if they only had one careful lady owner I don't think I could part with cash for a pair of used rubber *Directoires*. But *chacun à son goût*, I suppose.

Up to Level 4, the fantasy playroom. In one corner, a woman was whipping a man tied to a cross. She was wearing the outfit and expression of a particularly stern Victorian schoolma'am. Her waist measured around fifteen inches, a look corseting enthusiasts achieve through years of constriction. Unlike the half-hearted whippings I had seen in the past, Ma'am was really giving it what for and I feared, that from the force of her exertions, the top half of her body would snap away from the bottom half at any second. Like a golfing pro, she selected her tool from a caddy, cogitating over which instrument was best for which putt. A middle-aged public schoolgirl with full beard and pot belly was delighted by the teacher's expertise and, raising his pleated skirt, he pulled down his navy blue knickers and threw himself over a bench in squirming anticipation. The schoolmistress didn't disappoint. In fact, she drew blood. Ben tried to edge past her flailing tawse on his way to the bar, but she cornered him and smartly planted one on his behind, saying, 'I'm generous. Oh, yes, I'm very generous'.

The toilets were a hive of activity. I stood waiting with Dominic outside one very tiny cubicle. Condom wrappers had fallen out under the door and the groans coming from within suggested that somebody was relieving more than a bladder in there. I could also hear the sound of whipcracks coming from the same lock-up and guessed that, as small as the convenience was, there was obviously enough room to swing a cat. The cubicle next to it was similarly occupied. After a while, a woman emerged, followed a couple of minutes after by a sheepish-looking man. It was clear that the two had never met before in their lives.

I went into the cubicle accompanied by Dominic (it was still bloody difficult getting in and out of the dress unaided) and tried to do my business whilst ignoring the footprints on the toilet seat. Realising that when we left, the next person coming in would think the footprints were mine, Dominic decided to brazen it out.

He opened the door with a bang, cracked Doris and said, rather loudly, in front of the waiting queue, 'And let that be a lesson to you, bitch'.

With my hand over my face, I followed him out, ignoring the sympathetic looks I was getting from the queue. Outside, I bumped into the owner of the footprints and asked him what he had been doing in there.

'Oh, it was fantastic!' he said.

'Were you screwing?'

'Oh no. She was posing for me while I wanked. She wouldn't allow me to come until she had counted to five. It was brilliant.'

Back outside Ben had discovered that the school-mistress wasn't as generous as she claimed, and after giving him a free taster Ben got the feeling she was trying to negotiate a price to continue with her services. Needless to say Ben didn't feel that anybody should have to pay for their education and she had returned her attention to the possibly more financially rewarding blood-spattered rump of the St Trinian's girl.

However, the teacher's enthusiasm had started some-thing in the playroom, as now there were more whips going than at the Grand National. The piercing videos had been replaced by straightforward porn to which one Japanese man in a leather pouch was masturbating enthusiastically. I noticed that he didn't leave it alone all evening and could only hope that he put a hot poultice on it before he went to bed. As we were making for the dance-floor, a woman stopped me and gave me a flyer.

'We're raising Pan next week and you've simply got to come,' she said, then was away with the fairies.

On the dance-floor, my thigh boots soon filled up with sweat. Sitting down to drain them off, I was joined by the world's best dad from Submission. He was looking rather forlorn as his wife had disappeared with another man. I barely had chance to commiserate with him before being dragged off by a leatherdyke in a trench-coat for a twirl around the dance-floor. On one of my many revolutions, I saw Ben with his back to me, talking to Dominic. I noticed a white mark on the seat of Ben's suit and extricated myself from the grasp of the trench-coat for a closer look. The strain borne by a medium suit from an XL bum had taken its toll, for the white mark was a square inch of Ben's buttock protruding through a rip in the rubber.

'I did feel a sudden change in pressure,' he said, shocked, 'but I just thought somebody groped me.'

Hurrying off to the toilets to assess the damage, he insisted that Dominic follow up in the rear to prevent any opportunists fingering the slit.

Waiting at the bar for them to come back, I got talking to a woman called Marie who was dressed as a leather version of the Little Dutch Girl. It transpired that Marie was something of a doyenne of the fetish scene, involved with running magazines and events. I seized on the chance of having some of fetishism's finer points explained to me. I asked her if it was just a sex thing.

'At a club like this,' she said, flicking back a wire-stiffened yellow plait, 'with about 700 to 1,000 people, maybe around 300 want sex and probably only half of those are in with a chance of getting it. For others, just looking is enough of a thrill.'

She felt that fetish clubs were more honest than ordinary clubs when it came to sex. 'You can't tell me people aren't trying to get off with each other in other clubs. Here, it's just more open, more in-your-face.'

Were the 150 who were getting it likely to be getting it SM style?

'Just because people are into the clothes, it doesn't mean they are into sado-masochism, although the two do tend to go together. But there are plenty of people at home in Laura Ashley frocks being whipped.'

And well they deserve to be. I wanted to know that if SM sex and fetishism were in many cases bed-partners, why did they stop people on the doors of clubs for looking too ordinary? Why, for instance, stop Ben for wearing jeans when, for all the bouncer knew, he could be a raging sadist?

Marie explained. 'The dress code is there because the clothes are a sign of commitment. We all look bloody stupid but nobody is going to laugh at anybody else. We're all vulnerable. Actually, that's not quite true. You do laugh at some people. Human sexuality is pretty comical and like most things, fetishism does have its fair share of trainspotters.' And to prove her point, the man with the nylon panties and studded belt walked by. He looked the type to loiter around train stations from time to time.

Marie scotched my belief that the fetish scene was a completely democratic one by admitting that there was a tier system with the trainspotters standing around their barbecues dressed in rubber talking about football at one end and quite exclusive private parties at the other. She said that there were mixed feelings on the scene about the Spanner case. Marie didn't feel that there should be laws preventing people from indulging in consensual SM activity, but she did think their behaviour was a little strange.

'I don't think there're too many people on the scene interested in having their arses scraped by an electric sander.'

As the subject turned to arses, Dominic emerged from the toilets bent double with laughter followed shortly after by Ben who was howling. Ben had tried to pull the hole around slightly so that he could see it and the back of the suit had came apart in his hands. He turned around to show us his not inconsiderable bum, now fully exposed to the elements. Although he was quite content to display a full moon for the rest of the evening, perhaps in hope of a chance meeting with an electric sander, he kept a close watch on the tear's inexorable move along his gusset. Mid-scrotum, he decided enough was enough and we left, passing Mark the Tranny who had a reluctant woman pressed up against the wall.

'You look saucy,' he said. 'Are you looking for action?'

Unfortunately, the collapse of Ben's suit didn't mean the end of our fetish experiences. We still had the tickets for the Boat Party. Ben briefly entertained the idea of kitting himself out in nautical neoprene, then thought better of it and settled for wearing Dominic's suit. Although both outfits had been marked medium, Dominic's actually seemed much smaller. Watching Ben get into it was not unlike seeing someone pull an arm-chair stretch cover over a sofa. For my own part, the red dress was on its way to an endurance record that Goodyear would have trouble matching. Meanwhile, Dominic took the precaution of packing his gas mask which he intended to use as a snorkel if the boat went down.

And so, armed with a packet of Quells, we queued along the Embankment to board the boat. Amazingly, Saucy Mark was not among the assembled crew but there was a whole galley-full of transvestites in French-maid outfits. One of the carrots to actually get us out for the evening was the fact that a meal was to be served during the voyage, though I wasn't too sure if Ben should eat anything while wearing Dominic's suit.

Most of the other people on the boat obviously viewed the meal as something of an enticement too, as the dining area was packed out. As we squeezed on to a table, everything suddenly went quiet. A screaming woman was dragged down the aisle by two men, one of whom was the pony-cart maker whom we had seen at the fetish

market. She was bound and gagged and then handcuffed to a pillar. The two men then produced a
selection of whips and set about her with vigour. I fancied that the two men were fetish customs officials and
they had caught her trying to smuggle a contraband
tweed two-piece on board. Whatever, when they finally
untied her, she had a big smile on her face. Watching
this drama played out, I hadn't noticed the boat casting
off.

As we cruised towards the Isle of Dogs, I went to the
bar where the incredibly straight bar staff seemed very
bemused by the night's duty they'd volunteered for. As I
was buying a drink, a member of the trainspotter element, in full regalia – grey leather bomber jacket, posing
pouch, slip-on shoes – stuck his tongue down my throat
and his hand on my breast. I kicked his shin which he
took as a come on and followed me back to the table to
ask me for a dance. Ben, as ever, was ready with the whip
and his lariat of a tongue. The trainspotter fled to the
poopdeck.

Settling down with the beers, I watched the trannies
in the galley messing around with some lettuce in a
bowl. Dinner looked far from ready. An old man in a
leather harness, accompanied by a vicar, came below
deck to check on its progress. The old man would have
looked fabulous had he remembered to take off his yel-
lowing string Y-fronts before putting on his harness.
Told that the lettuce was not yet ready, the two wandered back upstairs. This was when I noticed that the
vicar was wearing fishnet stockings. So maybe he was a
deaconess.

Sailing past Greenwich for the second time, the food
was still nowhere near ready. I distracted myself with the

sights outside the window and must say that London is very pretty at night. Occasionally, we would pull up alongside another pleasure cruiser and I would sink into my seat as another group of drunken revellers hurled insults and mooned at us. I had always hated the idea of going on a disco boat up the Thames. It always seemed so naff. And here I was doing it, and doing it in a rubber frock.

The trannies in the galley had lost much of their make-up by the time the food came out of the microwave. And what came out of the microwave was looking as bad as they did. This didn't seem to put any-one off and there was quite a scrum to get served. Ben had rather grandly bribed one of the waitresses to bring his meal over, but refused to reveal the exact nature of the bribe. As he ate, I swear I saw the straps of his outfit cut deeper into his shoulders.

I grew quite excited as the boat drew near the Embankment. Then my heart sank as we overshot the mooring and it was clear we were going for yet another circuit. The food over with, I wandered with Dominic to the upper deck while Ben went off to make his 'pay-ment'. Thirty or forty hardened fetishists were jiving away to 'Oh, Carol!' I sat down, not immediately realis-ing that the woman sitting next to me was performing oral sex on a man standing beside her. Before long, another woman was on her knees performing cunnilin-gus on woman A. Then woman C began playing close attention to B while being serviced by woman D and her husband.

'Would you like to do that?' I asked Dominic.

'Not to a Neil Sedaka record,' he replied.

I went to sleep. An hour or so later, I awoke and we

were nearing the Embankment again. Knowing we'd just go past it again and I'd be disappointed, I put my head down to go back to sleep. But it did stop.

It was over. Running down the gangplank, I felt that if I'd had anything else to wear, the red dress would have gone in the river. Dominic and Ben followed swiftly behind with a chorus of 'Never again!' Earlier in my enthusiasm, I had made plans to go to Weston-super-Mare to a fetish club called de Sade. A weekend of seaside and sadism had sounded so much fun. I cancelled those plans.

Chapter 6

NO BLUE KNICKERS
IN OXFAM

Ben read out the ad:

> The Muir Reform Academy. A real school for adult
> (twenty-one or over) girls, boys and 'boys who
> would be girls'. Don't miss a unique chance to go to
> school with your friends, meet new chums, relive
> your happiest times at school or rewrite the others.

'No!'

I couldn't see anything remotely sexy about reliving
my schooldays. I went to a very rough mixed-comp in
east London. Midnight feasts in the dorm with Binky
and Adele and unrequited Sapphic pashes for Matron it
was not. Which is not to say that there wasn't sexual
intrigue. But in our school that took the form of a book
run by the maths teacher on which of the third form
girls would fall pregnant by Summer Term. It was quite

a fair system. Even if your chosen runner managed to stay out of the maternity ward you were entitled to your stake back if she was spotted going into the VD clinic. Nobody ever lost money on that one.

Ben was persistent. 'I loved the Mallory Towers books. All those midnight feasts in the dorm with B—'

'I'm not doing it, Ben,' I said, interrupting his reverie.

'Come to think of it, I also used to love *Gilda of the Ice Cavern.* She was a skating superstar who got driven to international competitions in the back of a meat van. It had something to do with her not being able to do a Double Axle if the temperature went over freezing point.'

'What on earth are you on about?'

'I think you need to cast your net further afield. This rubber and swinging stuff is a bit obvious.'

'So you'd like me to get together with a bunch of middle-aged schoolboys and perform a nude "Face the Music" on Lea Valley Ice Rink?'

'It would have got Torvill and Dean the gold.'

'I'm not going back to school.'

'It's either that or the adult baby club . . .'

Faced with explaining away nappy rash at my next gynie, I wrote off to Miss Prim. As per, I was soon inundated with promotional literature. An introductory leaflet explained that the emphasis at the school was on discipline. It noted: 'A formal timetable, constant supervision and enforced adherence to strict rules, rapidly turns a random set of adult individuals from every walk of life into a group of school chums. They become absorbed in their studies and life in school, outside concerns forgotten.'

It went on to say that the Academy was Miss Prim's

dream, and as Headmistress, she alone controlled every aspect of its running. Somewhere in the background was her consort, Sir Guy Masterleigh, Chairman of the Governors and editor of the *Muir Journal.*

Along with the introduction, I received *The Rod Rack,* a catalogue of books, photo sets, tapes and instruments for all those corporal punishment fans. In the literary section there was, *Half Naked She Obeyed, Anita's Smoking Bottom* (a sequel, I guessed, to *Anita's Smoking Beagle*), *The Romance of Chastisement, Sounds from the Study,* and *Stepmother Means Business. The Rod Rack*'s audio cassettes included a tape where a student gets more than she bargained for from Miss Prim. 'Hear her spanked, tawsed, caned and birched. Don't miss her gasp of horror on learning the penalty for lateness is one stroke per minute – she was seventy-five minutes late!'

The *Muir Journal* contained 'Stories From The Headmistress's Study' and 'Matron's Case Notes'. I flicked through a piece entitled 'Some Thoughts On Underpinnings By A Mature TV' and was disappointed to find no mention of the problems of subsidence. A Norwegian Old Boy had written in to say that 'punishment and humiliation are central items in the play on domination and submission. Many men and women enjoy being disciplined by a stern, dominant woman, for instance the all-powerful, strict schoolmistress.' And Miss Prim was certainly strict. There were pages and pages of her rules only to be capped off by a caveat warning that all rules were null and void when Miss Prim had PMT – 'Miss Prim is ready when she is ready.'

I also received the school prospectus which looked very official and included the words of the school song.

Sung to the tune of 'Onward Christian Soldiers' it had four verses, the first being:

> No more television, comic books and toys,
> No more late-night movies for the girls and boys,
> We must wear our uniform and obey the rule:
> New term starts tomorrow, we go back to school.
> Reading, writing, spelling and arithmetic,
> And if you're not careful, you will get the stick!

As with any good school, every prospective pupil was subject to an intensive interviewing and examination procedure. I rang the school and spoke to a man who I later found out was Sir Guy.

'Miss Prim is out shopping,' he said in a quavery voice. 'And she doesn't let me make appointments since I double booked her.' If Sir Guy thought Miss Prim something of a Tartar, he let nothing slip. He merely observed, 'When Miss Prim goes shopping, she goes shopping.'

Later in the day, after several attempts, I managed to get hold of the venerable headmistress. She sounded quite nice; but firm too. After some preliminaries, she asked, 'Have you got a school uniform?'

I meekly admitted my failure and promised to get one for the interview.

'Well don't go to too much expense as you might not get into the school. You can wear a gym-slip. But, by the way, all girls are interviewed as junior girls so you must wear long socks. Later you can progress to a senior girl. Have you ever been to this type of school before?'

'Er, no. But my partner and I have indulged in those type of fantasies.'

'General SM fantasies or school in particular?' she asked.

'Oh, a bit of both, you know.'

I racked my brains to come up with something more concrete but I couldn't. I sensed Miss Prim was less than pleased but she agreed to meet me in a café for a chat so we could check each other over. After that we would adjourn to her study for the interview proper.

'You do realise you'll be disciplined at the interview?'

So she *was* mad at me. 'How hard?' I asked, trying to keep the terror from my voice.

'Under severe for the interview. In fact, I have had interviewees that are disappointed. I've only had one who left after two strokes of the cane. Of course, everyone's idea of severe is different . . .'

For the pleasure of Miss Prim's administration, I had to pay a hundred pounds. She asked if my partner wanted to come too. I pointed out that at twenty pounds a stroke he might have to forgo the ecstasy this time. For the first time in our conversation Miss Prim brought a little sunshine into my life by saying that she would throw in my partner for the same price. So Gilda of the Ice Cavern would have to come with me. I was sure that an hour under Miss Prim's tutelage would soon knock the shine off his blades.

Unfortunately, our application to the local education authority for a school uniform grant was rejected and so we turned to the celebrated outfitters of many a public school child – Oxfam. Ben went for a symphony in polyester (blazer £2.19, shorts £1.25) while I made do with a beret, a blue pleated skirt and a short-sleeve blouse with the Midland Bank logo on it. We out-Buntered Bessie and Billy. Blinky and Addled and all of the girls of the

Lower Sixth Remove would chuck up their tuck with jealousy when they saw us. I was slightly panicked by not being able to find any knee-length socks and hoped Miss Prim had remembered to take her Evening Primrose oil.

The headquarters of the Muir Reform Academy were situated just on the border with Wales and we had to catch a nine o'clock train from Paddington. I got to the station at a quarter to with the warning of what had happened to the girl who was seventy-five minutes late very firmly on my mind. Ben wasn't there. As the minutes ticked away I grew more and more anxious. What could have happened to him? Maybe somebody had stolen his lunch money. Maybe he had wet himself. Maybe the joke was on me and he had no intention of turning up in the first place. As I boarded the train on my own I vowed that I would give his phone number to the biggest girl in the Remedial Fifth.

My mood wasn't helped by the fact that I was stone cold sober. A lady never drinks on her own before noon says Mrs Shirley Churchill (although for some reason she doesn't extend this to the bottle of Kahlua she keeps hidden in her flour bin) and I must admit the sight of a woman in her mid-thirties and a beret attacking a Stella six-pack in the buffet compartment of the 9 AM from Paddington would have been a sad one. So with my faculties completely intact, I worried myself stupid. The caning I could understand, after all over the last few months I had become quite handy myself in the CP department. But the thought of pretending to be a teenage schoolgirl all afternoon! How did Maureen from *Please Sir!* manage for all those years?

Miss Prudence Prim was waiting for me outside the station. I felt quite relieved when I saw her. She was a plump, bespectacled woman sporting a blonde curly perm, coral pink lipstick and immaculately manicured nails. Smartly turned out in a suit, she looked like a nice, middle-class, middle-aged mum. Softly spoken, she was not the sort of woman I could imagine being capable of inflicting too much pain. We went for a coffee so she could make sure I knew what I was letting myself in for and to check I wasn't from the *News of the World*. One of the Sunday tabloids had done an exposé on the school which had hurt her greatly. It was, she told me, like someone coming into her bedroom without being invited. Or someone coming into her study without knocking, I would imagine. She was very relaxed, which is more than could be said for me. I told her why Ben hadn't made it.

'If he was mine,' she said with sudden authority, 'he wouldn't sit down for six months.'

Miss Prim filled me in on the history of the Academy. Once merely a sexual hobby, her interest in schools became a full-time career after the collapse of her business six years ago. The Academy was held at various locations around the country and had over two thousand members dotted world-wide. Miss Prim told me several anecdotes about the members. One woman had phoned her asking if her husband was a member. Sadly, he had died without ever telling her about his secret schooldays, which was a shame because it had always been her fantasy too. Another wife regularly sent her husband to the Academy when he was getting on her nerves.

The facilities on offer at each school varied. Some

had proper dormitories, one had a playground with swings and seesaws, another a proper playing field where they held Sports' Day. For the life of me I couldn't see how one could derive a sexual frisson from an egg-and-spoon race. But, as Miss Prim was keen to point out, there was no actual sex at the Muir Academy, merely a fantasy fulfilled to take away and use sexually if that was your bent.

'If the boys get an erection,' said Miss Prim, 'I just ignore it. Some of the girls need to take cold showers. Oh, and Matron often has to change her knickers.'

I had dropped all thoughts of a Sapphic pash for Matron. She sounded like a sadistic nightmare, doling out cod liver oil and corporal punishment with equal abandon. Nevertheless, claimed Miss Prim, the boys loved her and often visited her at her home during the school holidays.

'Do you have a safe word with Ben?' she asked.

(This is a code word agreed between sub and dom to indicate that for the sub, the action has gone too far, as saying 'oh, no, please stop' will but inflame the committed sadist.)

'Judy Garland,' I replied knowledgeably.

The word on use at the school was 'pax'. And it was now time to see if I could hold back from using it.

As she drove us back to her house in her Volvo, Miss Prim made it clear that acting out the role was as important as the corporal punishment. On arrival, I was ordered into the bathroom to change into my full uniform. I caught sight of myself in the bathroom mirror and my nerve failed for a second. What was I doing with myself? More importantly, why wasn't Ben doing it with me? He was probably sitting at home at that minute with a box of Milk Tray, watching a video of *All That Heaven Allows* and, in between tears, laughing himself stupid at the thought of me over Miss Prim's knee.

I knocked on the Headmistress's door. She opened it in gown and mortar-board and ushered me in. It smelt like a schoolroom. A mixture of musty books, sweaty little boys and chalk. As my eyes darted about the room I avoided paying undue attention to Miss Prim's rod rack. The woman had a frightening arsenal at her disposal.

'Sit down, Churchill!' she commanded, the softly spoken voice completely gone.

'How old are you, girl?'

'Do you mean real or pretend, Miss Prim?'

'Well, what age do you think you are, girl?' Miss Prim was losing her patience already.

'Fourteen.' God, the waist band on my pleated skirt was tight.

Miss Prim then asked me to stand so that she could give my uniform the once over. She skimmed over the griffin logo on my blouse without a word. All seemed to be going well but then she asked to see if I was wearing my regulation blue knickers. Unfortunately, Oxfam had been all out and I was wearing a white tanga. I had barely lifted my skirt and I was straight over her knee, tanga down and six of the best with the palm of her hand.

'Pax!' I wanted to say but it came out as, 'Thank you, Miss Prim.'

I hoped Ben choked on a cracknel.

'Do you know why you've been sent to this school?' asked the Headmistress, completely unflustered from her exertions.

Because Ben had been a very sad little boy who sat at home reading Mallory Towers books while all the normal kids were out stealing supermarket trolleys and sniffing glue. 'Because I've been a bad girl, Miss Prim.'

'Yes, and do you know what corporal punishment is?' Illegal? 'Caning, Miss.'

'It's more than that, Churchill, it is any punishment of a physical nature. You will learn discipline here as well as humiliation,' she told me, sternly.

I felt a surge of defiance. Her cane could not humiliate me any more than the beret had done already.

Miss Prim then recited the school rules. I was to count every stroke of the cane I was given and if I miscounted she would start again. I was not to rub my backside or call out as this would, once again, mean repeating the punishment. I was not to move until I was told to and I had to thank her at the end of each punishment session. Then she pointed to the blackboard.

'Read this!' she barked.

'Four demerits equal six whacks of the cane.'

Which probably helps to break down one's cellulite, I consoled myself.

The entrance exam was a fiasco. The first test was English Literature and whenever I didn't know an answer I said *King Lear*. I said that Shakespeare's wife was called Annie. I forgot the name of *A Midsummer-Night's Dream* and said it was 'the one with the fairies in'. I cursed my secondary school for making us study the canon of Jacqueline Susann. I got six out of twelve wrong. Miss Prim brought out a gym shoe. Back down came my knickers and I was bent over my desk holding on to my chair. I prayed that my tit wouldn't get lodged in the ink well.

Thwack went Miss Prim's gym shoe six times.

'You've obviously been spending too much time behind the bike shed with the boys.'

If only she knew.

Mere mention of the next test filled me with dread. Home Economics. I tried desperately to remember four ways to serve a baked apple and how to remove Windowlene stains from an ironing-board cover. But Miss Prim had been right. We didn't have a bike shed at our school but we did have a bin room and I was under the impression that what I learnt there would keep a man far happier than knowing how to make a butterfly cup cake. But thanks to the grace of God, or at least the ghost of Elizabeth David, I scraped through with nine out of twelve. Had I not said that the principal ingredient of a Quiche Lorraine was Sainsbury's it would have been ten. Nevertheless, three were wrong and I was back over the desk having my bum tanned with a leather paddle. I don't know why I pulled my knickers up, I knew they were coming down again.

Sooner than I thought. Flushed with my cookery triumph I got cocky and made a big mistake. I forgot to thank Miss Prim for her troubles. Out came the tawse – a flat whip with a number of leather tails.

'Rude!' Swish. 'Disobedient!' Swish. 'Stupid!' Swish.

Raindrops on roses, I thought, remembering having once seen a naked Ben accidentally sit on a hot radiator. Though I wished him death, as Miss Prim swished, I was glad he wasn't there. He would have made me laugh and the punishments would have been more severe. Worse still, the swot would have probably got all the questions right. But it was jarring to think that had he been there, my punishment time would have been halved. As my buttocks began to glow, I thought about the time that Ben was run over outside of *No Sex Please We're British* and then, as he was lying in the road, punched by the driver for denting his fender. Whiskers on kittens, indeed.

Round three, the History Test, and Miss Prim wasn't even out of breath. Despite having History A level, I floundered. Eleven out of fifteen wrong. I certainly didn't know what started the English Civil War. Should Miss Prim be asking you at a future date it's apparently something to do with a woman throwing a chair at a Dean over the Common Prayer. The Headmistress seemed to have a sudden lapse in inventiveness and for my punishment I was back over her knee with her using her hand. Unfortunately, I miscounted just on the last stroke. She began again. I started to laugh, almost uncontrollably. Tears streamed down my face.

And still the CP kept coming. Somehow, throughout the afternoon I had gained four demerits. My knickers had whiplash from being jerked backwards and forwards so quickly. Over the desk once more, I gratefully received my caning. As she swished the cane behind me I felt faint. I had never been caned in my life before and by now my bottom was seared from an hour of her ministrations. I swore under my breath as I counted out the six blows, telling myself it would soon be over. It had become a battle of wits. I knew I could say 'pax' and it would stop, but I wouldn't give Miss Prim the satisfaction.

'Judy Garland!' I yelled by way of consolation.

As a final note Miss Prim asked me if I was going to write a letter to my previous school apologising for my past behaviour and promise to try harder at the Muir

Reform Academy. Saying no would have meant the birch but I was definitely tempted.

'Oh, yes, Miss Prim. Yes.'

To all at my former school,
I, Kitty Churchill, do hereby apologise for the bin room incidents, for excessively backcombing my hair, for hitting Carol Parsons of 4C in the mouth with a G-clamp, for my non-regulation knickers, for laughing till I peed when the deaconess fell off the stage during Harvest Festival, for locking Mr Blunden in the art cupboard and thus contributing to his eventual nervous breakdown and for robbing the sanitary dispenser blind. What can I say? I was crying out for attention and it was a shame that I had to go as far as I have to find it. If only you lot at the secondary modern had believed in Miss Prim's brand of tough love.

I took off my uniform and Miss Prim was waiting for me in the kitchen with tea and sympathy.

'Did you think your punishment was light, medium or severe?' she asked, removing the tea cosy.

Severe, I thought, but I knew that if I said that she would wonder why I went there in the first place. 'Medium. No sugar for me, thank you.'

Miss Prim played mum and told me that on the contrary my punishment had been very light. She said that I obviously had a low pain threshold and would write this down on my school card for the new term. We discussed the possible school days and weekends I could attend. I must say I was very tempted by the weekend girls-only (special girls allowed) school which placed particular emphasis on the 'feminine arts'. These included deportment, elocution and flower arranging. But thinking about what I could do to a handful of 'mums and a block of oasis, I decided that maybe it would be easier on my bum if I went for a one-day mixed school.

The train home was full of businessmen talking in very loud voices about budgets, product placement and managerial skills. As I sat, squirming from my bruises, I began to wonder about the task I'd set myself. I felt very removed from the normality around me. Then thinking about it further, I realised that the 'normal' businessmen sitting around me were probably doing the same things as me on a far more regular basis.

Ben was waiting for me when I got back home, claiming he'd missed the train as he'd been stuck on the tube. He insisted that I show him my bruises.

'So was it *All That Heaven Allows*?' I asked, pulling down my knickers for the nth time that day.

'*Magnificent Obsession*,' he replied. 'You want to put something on that.'

Chapter 7

WE'RE ALL BODIES UNDERNEATH

A couple of days after the interview, I was sitting on a ring cushion when the phone went. It was Adam from the Party Susan Club belatedly phoning me to check that I hadn't choked on my own vomit. It transpired that the party in Kensington had merely been a pre-med for the big op – a full-on swinging affair in a Gothic tower in the heart of the Kent countryside.

'It's going to be very special,' promised Adam. 'There's going to be a live show, prizes for the sexiest-dressed person, there's a Jacuzzi and a four-poster games room.'

I accepted his invite quickly and said goodbye, partly because I didn't want him to fill me in on the missing forty-five minutes I'd spent face down in his lap. The other reason was that Dominic had picked up the extension to listen in on the call.

'A four-poster games room, eh?' he said afterwards.

'I'm sure it means somewhere with a shove-ha'penny board and a few Mucha prints on the wall,' I said, shifting on my cushion.

Dominic wanted to come with me. He was excited by the idea of a naked romp in a National Trust Jacuzzi but I'm sure in his fantasy he didn't picture the other bathers as looking like the anaphrodisiac Adam and co. As that was exactly what Ben pictured the other bathers as looking like, he would have been only too happy to stand down as my consort. Dominic refused to believe my protestations about how hard the Party Susans had been hit by the ugly stick.

'Group sex is a big fantasy of mine,' he suddenly admitted.

'Ten minutes in the Jacuzzi with Wiggy would pop that particular balloon,' I said, picturing her in a floral bathing cap on top of him. 'You can't come. Believe me, I'm doing you a favour.'

Dominic didn't believe me and on the night of the party threw a bit of a wobbly about being left out, which made it all the more awkward for me to have to ask him if he'd drive down later in the evening to collect us.

So I wasn't in the best of moods on the way down to Kent and the fact that there was no bar on the train would have been the final straw had Ben not gone through his rucksack and found some miniatures which had been given to him by a grateful Qantas steward. I was thinking about the sexiest-dressed person competition. How could I not win it? Just having my own hair put me head and shoulders above most of the other competitors. So, although I was wearing an outfit that would have looked over cautious on a nun, I had the rubber dress in my handbag. Ben, still peeved that I'd insisted he come instead of Dominic, hadn't even bothered to wash for the evening so at the very least I had to beat him.

We were told to meet the other party guests in a village pub. Arriving half an hour early, it suddenly occurred to me that we had no idea what the people we were going to be meeting looked like. The trouble with being in a small pub in Much Hampton on the Mind, on a Saturday night, was that everybody was dressed for sexcess. With only a finite number of available farmers, the women had to take the hard sell approach. Therefore, no hemline could be hiked too high, no neckline plunged too low. The acres of flesh outnumbered the acres of lycra by ten to one and stilettos were wielded in every colour as long as it was white. How could we sort out the swingers from the merely cheap? Ben refused point blank to go up and ask anybody.

'What would I say?' he asked. 'Excuse me, sir, but at some point this evening am I likely to be indulging in some heavy-duty frottage with your lady wife?'

The white stilettos were the first sign that something strange had happened between London and Much Hampton. Somewhere along the line we had slipped into the Twilight Zone and time seemed to be working backwards. Sipping a Rum and Pep, I ignored the exhortations from the DJ to join in the Rowing Song. The music slipped backwards through the seventies and I'm sure, just before Esther and Abi launched into 'Cinderella Rockerfella', I heard the couple at the next table discussing the three-day week. Where were the other swingers? Unless Wiggy jumped up on the bar and did the splits over the optics, I could see us spending the evening discussing the fuel crisis, saying no to Europe and wondering if Ruby would ever learn the secrets of Mrs Bridges' duff. As I tried to work out how much a tanner was in new pees, a woman dressed in a school uniform walked into the bar. Since she had probably borrowed the uniform off her granddaughter, I knew that I had found a swinger.

The pub was soon swarming with them. (I should never have worried about not being able to spot a swinger as there is definitely a uniform. Women who have changed hands more times than the Olympic flame wear a look of bitter experience. The men do wear white shoes and though the age of the Medallion Man may be long gone, there is still a gap in their chest tans where their krugerrands used to be. The swinging woman has a root lift; the swinging man has his hair pubicly permed, making him one big prick.) There were a couple of familiar faces. The petite brunette had been there all the time but I hadn't been able to see her over the top of the bar. Adam turned up last, still Moira-less. We left the pub *en masse* and followed Adam through the village in a crocodile, like some obscene school outing. Still, at least one woman looked the part.

We turned off the main road and found ourselves in a field in complete darkness. Somebody was flashing a torch in the distance and I could just about make out the outline of the tower against the night sky. As we got closer, we were told to keep quiet as the other tower residents were definitely not swingers. For a while, there was only the creak of a leatherette mini-skirt to be heard and the occasional curse as another spike heel went into a cow pat. Once inside, we were told which areas of the tower were out of bounds and shown where to change if we needed to. I needed to. With the competition as it was, the sexiest-dress prize was going to be a walk over.

Getting around the tower meant passing through entrances sometimes no more than four foot in height. Only the brunette could pass through unhindered. In the kitchen the party fare seemed above par for the Party Susan brigade but the drink was still in the Sarson's league. Ben went to open our own wine and, in his nervousness, managed to snap the corkscrew in half. It was an omen. And I didn't listen.

We moved into the living-room or what was probably The Great Hall. It was a circular room with heavy stone walls, a walk-in fireplace and real animal skins scattered across the floor. You would have thought that the air would have been heavy with sexual expectancy, but the snatches of conversation I heard from other people were rather mundane. These people, when asked, would invariably say that the reason they took up swinging was boredom and yet swinging seemed to bore them too.

'Didn't see you at the Ealing party last Saturday,' said one woman lifelessly to another.

'Couldn't find a baby-sitter,' she sighed back.

The women obviously saw each other week in, week out. They had come to the point in their marriages where, to get a new dishwasher, they had to put out for six boring men instead of just one. Realising they'd been duped, they'd switched off. They were dead behind the eyes.

Not that Ben was exactly the life and soul. He sat on a sofa, kicking the head of a snake skin and refusing to be drawn into conversation with anybody. I got chatting to a man, Billy, who recognised me from the hotel. It took a few minutes for it to dawn on me that he was the man who had brought me the wine when I was sitting on the toilet. Billy introduced his girlfriend Sabina, who, at nineteen, was a good twenty years younger than him. I asked him why he'd joined the club.

'We wanted a bit of excitement.'

Though the response was entirely expected, it made me angry. Here was a none-too-attractive man pushing forty with a very beautiful teenage girlfriend, moaning about the lack of excitement in his life. When was enough enough for some people?

Sabina added, giggling, 'It's a bit of variety.'

If she wanted change, I wanted to tell her, then change Billy for something with a few less miles on the clock. The conversation was cut short by all the lights being turned out. I joined Ben on the sofa. As the room grew quiet, he began to laugh.

At one end of the room, there was a small stage. Suddenly, entering from behind the arras, came Adam, dressed as the Grim Reaper. Ben laughed louder.

'Quiet, quiet,' the Grim Reaper roared, waving his scythe in Ben's direction. He made a welcoming speech and then added, 'There are ghosts in this tower. Tonight, before the celebrations can commence, we must first pay three forfeits to appease their restless spirits.'

A shiver went down my spine. It wasn't the ghosts; I knew that forfeits meant party games . . .

I was right. For game one, the Grim Reaper selected a woman from one side of the room and a man dressed in battle fatigues from the other. A black bin-liner was brought out and the Reaper informed them that they were to get inside and swap underwear. The couple were blindfolded and the bin-liner was then swapped for a clear plastic sheet. It wasn't much of a game as the woman wasn't wearing any knickers. I felt for her. There's been the odd wash day when I've had to go out knickerless but you'd think she would have made a special effort for a party. She could have just sponged down the crotch on an old pair.

As Grim pointed his scythe around the room to select the contestants for game two, Ben and I sank back into the sofa. I would have been more willing to go with the Reaper had he been the real thing. He picked three men and three women who were each given a party trick to perform. If their performance made any of the others laugh, the laugher had to forfeit an item of clothing. The fact that none of them undid so much as a button on their duffel coats should give you some idea of the level of hilarity this game provoked. Even Ben stopped laughing. One woman had to simulate intercourse with the aid of a three-foot inflatable penis, two men had to have a cock fight with dildoes and another did some kind of lion taming act of which I lost the plot completely. I seem to remember that a blow-up doll featured in the action too. She was the only one who looked remotely turned on.

I wasn't really watching the game too closely as I was trying to get an answer out of Sabina as to what she was doing with somebody like Billy. He misinterpreted my interest and offered Ben and me a lift back to London – no strings, of course. Which was a shame because the only way he would have been able to get me to have sex with him would be by tying me up first.

The Grim Reaper had warned that as the games progressed, more and more couples would have to become involved in the action. When he announced that he

needed five couples for the third game, I suddenly
wished I'd dropped my drawers in the bin-bag.
Fortunately, the others were such, if you pardon the
expression, eager beavers. The couples were swapped
around and the five men made to stand in a line with
their underwear around their ankles. The women were
then told to give the men an erection without using
their hands or mouths. As none of them were versed in
the erotic art of 'bagpiping' (just think about it), *coitus à
mamilla* was the only option available and bosoms were
bouncing like Space Hoppers. To surprisingly little
effect. Not a man was left standing. These people were
living out their fantasies and yet nobody was remotely
turned on. They weren't excited, I wasn't excited. Why
didn't everybody put their clothes back on so we could
all go home?

   The game was only brought to a head by one woman
giving it, and the recipient struggled wearily to half-mast.
Adam reappeared on the stage, still wittering on about
the ghosts. As a further appeasement, a woman was prepared to offer herself up as a sacrifice. And sacrifice she
certainly did. Beforehand she'd sacrificed her pubic hair,
during she sacrificed her knickers, and afterwards it
became pretty clear that she'd completely sacrificed her
integrity. She was an attractive woman in her late twenties
and was an erotic performance artiste. She selected one
balding man, pushed him to his knees and secured a
dog lead around his neck. She slipped behind the arras
and reappeared wearing a black party-size strap-on dildo.
Still on all fours, the dog's trousers were taken down and
she stroked between his cheeks with her plastic pipi.
Rather naively, I assumed that the Party Susan club had
just hired a rather enthusiastic Kiss-A-Gram. It took me a

while to realise that she was actually Linda, the party hostess. As she simulated buggery (or was it simulated bestiality?) her husband and our host, Darryl, looked fit to burst with pride.

For her next act, she lay totally naked on the stage with her legs in the air at ten to two, giving the crowd an excellent chance to study her topiary. She'd done a very good job but as I moved forward on the sofa to check for stubble rash, she obscured her entrance with the first in a long line of phoney phalluses. I looked at Darryl. 'That's my girl!' said the look on his face. The woman could have been a demonstrator at the Ideal Home Exhibition, such was her professionalism. As the dildoes upped in girth, she maintained her synchronised-swimming smile and sent her legs to quarter to three. Darryl's ecstasy knew no bounds when, dispensing with what must have surely been a traffic cone, for her finale, she selected two men from the crowd and entreated them to the oral delights of her front and back bum. This blew the crenellations off Darryl's turret. I was amazed to see that her exertions had left no trace on her vagina. She still had a snap like a mousetrap on her pubococcygea.

I noticed three black men standing at the back of the audience and went over to them. I mention their colour because the swinging scene seems to be a mostly white affair. They told me they were nurses and I really felt for them. They said they'd been invited by Darryl and were a little bit shocked by what was going on. When Darryl came over and said enigmatically to one of them, 'Are you still prepared to go through with the act?' I was a little confused. Were we going to have a first-aid demonstration?

The show in the Great Hall had finished. But, said Adam, there was more. He led the party down another of the tower's stairwells and into the master bedroom. The room was in semi-darkness and we fumbled our way, feeling for chairs that had been placed around a king-size bed. We were in the four-poster games room and there was definitely no sign of the shove-ha'penny board. The lights went down completely and then went up again to reveal Linda spreadeagled on the bed atop a satin sheet, exercising her pelvic floor muscles. Lord, that woman had worked hard for the party. I hoped Darryl would let her off picking up the beer cans afterwards.

She wasn't on her own on the bed for long. Very soon, two of the 'nurses' appeared in the bedroom, naked and rubbing their thermometers. I'd been so naive. The nurses took turns mounting Linda with ne'er a condom in sight. Occasionally, one of the men would hop off the bed and disappear behind a screen to restore his erection. Why these sudden attacks of modesty, I don't know. Ben was irate.

'It's so bloody racist,' he hissed. 'The black studs servicing the white mistress.'

Around the room, many of the men were fumbling in their trousers but I don't think they were looking for the phone number of the CRE. Pretty soon, Ben was one of the few men left not pulling his pud. During a breather, one of the nurses came and sat next to me.

I voiced Ben's objections. 'Don't you think there's an element of racism about this?'

'I don't know what you're talking about,' he replied.

Far be it from me to be a patronising liberal. I changed my tack. 'Why don't you use a condom? Don't you worry about HIV?'

'Don't depress me,' was his considered reply.

And that, to be honest, was about as deep as anyone at the Party Susan Club went. It was just there, they did it and didn't ask any questions. Well, if you can't beat 'em, join 'em, I thought, smoothing down my dress for the sexiest outfit competition, trying to ignore the fact that I'd just noticed a video camera on the bedroom wall.

It was a cattle market and only one cow was going to win. I stood in a line with five other women and stowed all of my feminist principles. The winner was to be judged by the amount of applause they received. The response to the first woman, the petite brunette, befitted her restricted stature. 'Pity that Ladybird hasn't introduced a lingerie line,' I smirked to myself. I was next. I struck a couple of lubricious poses in my latex and Ben barked appreciatively. The rest of the crowd were pretty lukewarm. I was aghast. When it came to the woman next to me, the crowd went wild. She was topless with a couple of chains draped across her breasts and wearing silver panties underneath, and get this, a regular pair of twenty denier American Tan tights. The rest of the competitors went for nothing. As she accepted her prize, I turned to her and said, in the spirit of Miss World, 'If I'd known all I needed to do to win was get my tits out I would have done it'.

She needed that bottle of Liebfraumilch more than I did.

It was coming up to the time I'd arranged for Dominic to pick us up, when I had an idea. If Dominic were to actually see what was happening there, I was sure that it would help to convince him that he was better off out of it. It was a bit of a risk. For all I knew, he could find the sight of Miss Sexiest Dress standing there in her hose the last word in wet dreams.

Chancing that he wouldn't, I found Darryl and told him that Ben and I had recently begun having a regular threesome with another man, who was at this very moment waiting in his car in the village to meet us, and could we invite him to the party. Ever the congenial host, Darryl agreed and showed Ben and me back to the main road, offering as he did so to photograph me for a fetishwear magazine.

'So many of my models hate wearing rubber,' he said. 'You obviously love it.'

I nearly said yes just to spite the woman in the tights, then it clicked. Linda and Darryl weren't merely enthusiastic amateurs. Neither were the nurses. They were all pros. I am shocked at my level of naivety sometimes. Here were a group of people willing to show their innards at the drop of a dildo and when Darryl had told me, just prior to asking me to be a model, that he was in the video business, I honestly thought he meant something like Blockbuster's. I've a lot of my mother in me. Her idea of a dirty video is not dusting her Betamax.

Walking back to the village, I told Ben that I was worried by the video cameras. 'I don't want to appear in a porn video, Ben,' I said.

'It would make a change from all those shoplifting ones you've been in,' he replied, spotting Dominic's car parked in a lay-by.

When he saw us, Dominic immediately resumed moaning about being left out and then looked completely horrified when I told him that he could come back to the tower with us in the guise of the *trois* in Ben and mine's *ménage*.

Returning to the tower, we made for the bedroom and I saw that my concern about the video camera had been right. Five people were naked on the bed under the camera's watchful eye which broadcasted their activities via a large screen TV in the corner. The wankers were out in force too and practically everybody was naked. We tried to seek refuge in the bathroom only to find Darryl and Linda and four of their closest friends enjoying the Jacuzzi.

'Come on in,' said Linda.

'I couldn't possibly,' I replied. 'The latex is the only thing that's holding me in.'

Linda was a philosopher. 'Don't worry about that, we're all bodies underneath.'

I couldn't think of any other excuses. Dominic had to pull me out of the dress.

'Check for video cameras,' I whispered. 'I don't want to end up on *You've Been Framed.*'

'And you too,' said Linda to Ben and Dominic. The boys looked at each other helplessly and undid their trousers.

Ben and I had had the chance to numb ourselves slightly with alcohol. But as Dominic was driving he had to stay completely sober and as he climbed into the Jacuzzi you could almost see his group-sex fantasy fly right out the window. The water was hot and the conversation strained. Every time I moved a hand or a foot, it brushed up against something unspeakable. Ben was smoking furiously over the other side and to Linda's complete horror was letting his fag ash drop into the water. You didn't need to be Desmond Morris to work out what his non-verbal communication was saying.

'Well, it is quite dirty in here,' I said by way of compensation, pointing at the tide marks.

'That's not dirt,' glowered Linda. 'I've been scrubbing all day.'

'My, it's hot in here,' I said, lifting my scalded nipples out of the water. All around me rhubarb-coloured penises were floating on the surface and, I fancied, panting for breath. I'd have been less worried swimming with garter snakes.

'Ooh, they're sexy,' said Linda, pointing to Dominic's tattoos. 'Who are you?'

'I'm having a mange-tout with these two,' he said, pointing at Ben and me.

Linda seemed unsure as to why Dominic felt the need to share his vegetable secrets and there was an uncomfortable silence. Eventually, this was broken by the man sitting opposite me making a few penis jokes.

'My, it's hot in here,' said Dominic and I simultaneously.

Dominic shot up, got out of the tub and wrapped himself in a towel. I did the same and we left the bathroom. Strangely, Ben didn't follow on.

The stone floor was cold on our feet as we wandered from room to room. In the basement we found an ersatz dungeon with a primitive rack. And to my delight, Miss Sexiest Dress was tied up on it. The temptation to turn the handle another notch and say 'How's that for your tits?' was great but I resisted.

'Would you like to sleep with her?' I whispered to Dominic.

'Where's the novelty value in having sex with another woman who's kept her tights on?' he said to me pointedly.

We returned to the master bedroom and Dominic admitted that he was completely freaked out by the orgy going on around us. He'd been expecting a little more discretion from the participants, though God knows why when so many breakfasts over the past few weeks had been interrupted by the arrival of Party Susan Polaroids.

'It's not the *sex* in group sex that bothers me,' I said, watching the cavorting on the bed. 'It's the *group*.'

As I said this, Ben reappeared, still nude.

'Why didn't you get out of the Jacuzzi when we did?' I asked.

'I was trying to get Darryl's toe out of my arse,' he said.

Dominic went off to get us a drink while we sat down in the bedroom and watched the TV. It may seem a little odd to watch a TV broadcasting something which was happening live a few feet away but watching it on a screen gave it a more palatable distance. Suddenly I felt a hand tweaking my nipples. I looked up to see the bald headed 'dog' with his other hand stuck up a woman's skirt. He obviously thought my breasts were detachable as he was trying his damnedest to pull one of them off. Ben realised what was happening and wrestled my breast out of the dog's paw. A naked nurse came and sat down beside us. Apparently, things had hotted up in the Jacuzzi after Ben had got out.

'Damn!' I said none too convincingly, rubbing my aching nipple.

'I want to go with her again,' said the nurse, pointing to a fortyish blond who was being seen to by two men on the bed. 'She's dynamite.'

Unfortunately, the woman decided that she'd had enough for one night and moved off the bed and got dressed. The threesome hadn't been alone. What from the TV screen, I had taken to be a bump in the duvet was, in fact, my little friend sitting on the face of her regular partner. What she did next was obscured by Ben appearing on the TV screen.

'God, it does put five pounds on you,' said Ben, watching himself, ignorant to the fact that I was now rubbing the nurse's penis.

Dominic's timing was immaculate. Coming back with the drinks he immediately noticed my French polishing. 'Home! Now!' said Dominic, indignantly.

'He put it in my hand. What was I supposed to do with it?' I asked, letting go. 'You just don't appreciate the rigours of research.'

As Ben went off to retrieve our clothes, Dominic glared while I gave it another quick rub for luck. The nurse didn't seem to mind too much when I stopped. He went off and flattened the bump in the mattress.

Ben came back from the bathroom and threw our clothes at us. He was apoplectic.

'I can't get to my knickers,' he snarled. 'Some fat man is sitting on them having a wank.'

Once I had my clothes on, I felt rather overdressed. More people had arrived since I last looked and now there were around sixty people there in various stages of intercourse. As Ben was pulling on his shoes, still muttering about losing his Calvins, Adam came over to us. It was the first time I had seen him since the party games.

'Can I come and join in your conversation?' he asked. 'Nobody else wants to talk to me.'

'No, we're having a row,' said Dominic and Adam scurried off.

Poor Adam. It was pretty clear that nobody had lifted his habit all night.

There was no-one to show us back to the road. Ben was still cursing me for taking him to the tower and therefore losing him his underpants. He strode into the darkness in a temper and promptly fell, head first, into a ditch. Dominic dragged him out and we returned to the tower to enlist the aid of a torch. Dominic was furious too, but not about my little diversion with the nurse. His manhood had been questioned and found wanting. He'd had the chance to act out his fantasy and it had terrified the life out of him. Walking back to the car I had both of them whingeing in unison.

'Just wait for the TV make-over,' I thought.

Chapter 8

ONLY A LETTER
AWAY!*!

The tower party left its mark and a certain amount of
desensitisation was setting in. Sex was beginning to be
a chore, something to be saved for work. None of us
actually did it any more. Ben claimed that he didn't
mind that he'd not had an orgasm in weeks but said
that he had started to make a macramé plant pot
holder as he still hadn't quite worked out what to do
with his hands.

One evening, coming back from a rare, non-sexual
and much needed night out with the girls, I found
myself strangely in the mood. Quietly letting myself into
the house, I crept up the stairs pulling off my clothes to
surprise Dominic with the offer of my body. But it was
me that was surprised. I caught him in his office,
engaged in a disgusting vice that until that moment in

our relationship I'd had no idea he practised. He was playing a computer game. I tried gesturing at my bare but wilting bosoms in a lewd manner but to no avail. Dominic had totally embraced this new sexless period of our lives and had become an anorak. Worse still, I didn't really care.

I told Ben about this sorry event the next day. To illustrate the point that I had at one time been a fully-fledged sexual being I dug out an old photo of myself taken by an ex-boyfriend. In it I was posing as a sexy secretary, sitting topless on a kitchen stool, wearing sexy specs and white stilettos, poring over a copy of *War and Peace*.

'I'm shocked,' said Ben.

'See, I told you,' I replied. 'I was really into sex at one point.'

'No, I'm shocked that you've read Tolstoy.'

And so this sad, sexless state persisted for a while. A week or so later, I was sitting in the bath, flicking through the small ads in the fetish magazine *Skin Two*, and it slowly dawned on me that I had been humming a Carpenters' medley for the past fifteen minutes. This gave me a clue as to what was causing our malaise. Spontaneously bursting into 'Yesterday Once More' was my subconscious's way of telling me that my life was getting too dark. One more set of handcuffs, one more *ménage à trois*, and I would go over the brink. Then I spotted an ad which I felt might lift my spirits. It read: Enhance – the organisation for those interested in loving and gentle eroticism.

On receiving the first of many letters from Enhance, it became clear that Gillian, the club director, was a very special woman, a woman with a heavy duty secretary fetish. Gillian's lime high-lighter pen ran wild over her missives until what was not high-lighted became more important than what was. Her punctuation was something of a marvel and I'm sure a police psychologist would say that it showed the hallmarks of a budding serial killer. She! was! lavish!! with! exclamation marks!!! and her usage of the asterisk had me fruitlessly scouring the bottom of the page looking for footnotes that the minx felt were unnecessary to supply.

Still, I was enthusiastic. The chance of some loving and gentle eroticism had me hooked. According to Gillian, Enhance had, for over a decade, dedicated itself to promoting safety, responsibility and common sense in the enjoyment of dressing for pleasure, adult games and fantasies. Membership, she continued, was selective and should be beneficial to those who felt isolated by virtue of their particular interests (Alma Cogan fans?) and allowed prompt, personal response on all matters and help with advice to widen their horizons (where to buy a Rosemary Clooney album?) and 'play safe' in their private lives. The club **WELCOMED** (the word high-lighted almost to the point of obliteration) applications 'from* responsible, mature, couples, singles *be they; "normal", bi, homo, transsexuals, or transvestites of either sex – it matters not! We are people-conscious and Gillian is always just a letter away.' Just a letter away from her next victim, I began to think.

Despite the generosity of her welcome, it was at no point clear what it was that I was actually joining. Although, in retrospect, the fact that Gillian chose to advertise in *Skin Two* should have given some clue as to her idea of loving and gentle eroticism. At the bottom of the first letter was an offer for a copy of the Enhance Newsletter Special Issue (£3) and a note that I needed to pay £2 for an application form. I did so and, by return of post, I received my second letter. I could tell it was from her even before I opened the envelope. I could smell the high-lighter pen. Again, in this letter, Gillian extended a warm welcome to all-comers and reminded me that she was only a letter away (and getting closer all the time, I feared). She delighted in the fact that 'We always circulate on time'. The 'we' bit had me wondering. Gillian said that all applications were considered at monthly staff meetings. There were others! Were they the bodies of those from whom she was no longer a letter away, propped up around the table of the Enhance boardroom?

This thought brought out the Jodie Foster in me. I scoured the special-issue newsletter to see where Gillian, or, as I had come to know her, 'The Punctuator', would strike next. There were about thirty photocopied pages featuring 'Gillian's free-wheeling editorial', murky reproed photographs of nipple piercing, a transvestite in latex and yet again, a woman who looked suspiciously like Ben's Aunty Josie, modelling her bondagewear alongside ladies of a similar bent. It was the same old, same old. My hopes of a loving and gentle eroticism now lay in tatters. But I had to continue. Josie could be at risk.

The adverts in the newsletter did nothing to dampen my mounting apprehension:

Pot luck! First come first served! Ladies' wigs just £2 each including P&P.

Play *safe!* The ultimate in personal protection against infection, etc. our 'Coverall' (including scrotum).

*Knickers!** Clearing wardrobe. All kinds and colours, some as new. State your preferences . . . Or one pair 'worn' as requested and letter confirming the conditions you request.

So the bodies in the boardroom, were scalpless, ball-less and knickerless. This woman was a monster.

In her introduction, Gillian apologised that the newsletter may have missed out on some special interest areas. I glanced at the contents list which ran the gamut from nappy wetting to slavery with, I must say, a disturbing fixation on The Art of the Enema. What was there left that Gillian could possibly tell us? What a suitable replacement for a nice Chianti could be for those on a budget? One thing Gillian did neglect, despite her constant high-lighted exhortation 'BE NICE TO EACH OTHER! GIVE PLEASURE!', was how the hell does one administer an enema in a loving and gentle fashion? Dear 'Constipated and Vanilla, Crouch End' – remember, Gillian is only an exclamation mark away*!*. (I learnt subsequently that there is, in America, a group actually called 'Gentle Enemas'.)

Gillian hinted at the delights that the full membership of £25 could bring. Aside from the ads and the editorial, she also offered a confidential purchasing service for toys and props/special equipment that might be difficult to otherwise obtain. I took this to mean advice on where to buy a house with a fifteen-foot well in the cellar or one of those lovely coffee-table books on shrapnel wounds. Her staff, she said, have considerable practical and research experience. It was a pity, therefore, that they were probably no longer breathing.

From an article on safe bondage, I got the feeling that Gillian was wrestling with her conscience. She was disparaging about the term SM, feeling that the practices described in many fetish magazines could be harmful and did not relate to *reality*. She preferred the term ET which stood for erotic torments. In a touchy, feely manner, she laid down the basics for ET: the dominant party should have experienced the treatment to be used on the slave, the subject's state of health should be known (particularly if treatment is to be prolonged). Use a code word to signal distress. (Where the subject is gagged a push-button operating a light or bell can be used.) Keep a sharp knife and metal-cutting tools to hand. (Locks have been known to jam, keys get lost, etc.) A pair of shears is useful for straps, etc. 'It is better,' she noted, 'to destroy expensive equipment than lose a valuable and devoted slave and face the coroner!'

She continued. 'Before a session the subject should remove any dentures, contact lenses, etc. Breathing should be checked. Never restrict the neck. Do not attach suspension (even slack) rope, chains to the collar of a vertical subject. They might topple over and hang/break their neck! Beware of excessively tight restraints – an interrupted blood supply can maim or kill!' She never actually said, 'Dear Reader, learn from my experience,' but I think that could have been what she meant. I read between the lines. Gillian wanted redemption. I had to join Enhance and save her.

Another reason for joining was an intriguing letter

from Mrs B.D., Rochester. She began, 'A number of years ago, feeling a little frustrated, I gave in to my hairdresser's suggestion and changed my hair colour with a Titan rinse, though I feared the result might be a bit "brassy".' To her amazement, the hairdresser went off and reappeared wearing a black leather trenchcoat and said to Mrs B.D., Rochester, 'This is the type of thing that goes with your hair now. You'll feel totally different.' The hairdresser then lent her a black shiny plastic mac to thrill her timid husband and the rest, as they say, was history. The couple now had a full range of erotic clothes, shoes and toys. Their sex life had improved so much that it had led to several job promotions for Mr B.D., Rochester. That settled it. Joining Enhance was now an imperative. I had to find out what a Titan rinse was.

I filled in the application and put Ben down as my partner. If we had to go to a mortuary, only he could identify Josie from her nipple rings. On the form we had to declare that we would not be offended/perverted in any way by joining Enhance and tick off a list of our pursuits. We ticked off everything – Bi, Sub, Dom, Leather, Rubber, PVC, Bondage, Water Sports (Just tell me, what exactly is the sporting element of micturition?), Anal, Bondage and Piercing. There was no telling where Josie would wash up.

I was on tenterhooks. Acceptance was not guaranteed. Would Gillian accept us? In fear of rejection, I spent many sleepless hours pacing up and down my office, searching through copies of *Hair International* for a clue to the Titan rinse. Nothing. When, one morning, the postman finally delivered a letter with that familiar chemical tang, I was ecstatic. I tore it open. Gillian was writing to allay our fears that we had been forgotten. We were in luck!! she said. The staff meeting was only a few days away and she couldn't see any problems with our being accepted. I would have thought that the corpses on the board would by dint of decay have great difficulty in blackballing anybody. The arrival of that letter sent me to fever pitch. The anticipation was unbearable. Fortunately, I only had to wait for the second post. '*Congratulations!!!!' said the letter. 'Your welcome* awaits!' We were in.

To be honest, I wasn't quite sure *what* we were in and, as the letters from Gillian suddenly dropped off, I began a correspondence with another woman of a similar bent in the hope that she could throw some light on Gillian's psychological make-up. The woman was Deborah Ryder, chair of The Lady O Society, a group dedicated to promoting the activities of the submissive woman.

Deborah's introduction letter gave a quick resumé of herself. 'I am forty-six (though I don't look it, I have always taken care of my appearance, especially complexion), slim, brunette, I live with two lovely cats. I am a member of Cats Protection League and other animal welfare charities. I am disabled (multiple sclerosis) and cannot walk much . . . It also means that my Master has to be more merciful than he used to be, but I still get some quite spectacular stripes. As I have said before, subs learn the real meaning of the word trust. Actually, I have the right temperament to be disabled – extremely lazy. I used to pay a cleaning lady, now she is paid by the Department of Social Services.'

Reading thus far it became clear that Deborah was a woman every bit as complex as Gillian. One could only imagine what it would be like to bring these two

Amazons together. Then again, if you've seen *Whatever Happened to Baby Jane?* you probably don't need to imagine it at all.

Deborah wrote a long piece called 'Writing Sado-Masochistic Pornography: A Woman's Defence'. Deborah believed that masochists and sadists are born, not made. 'I believe that our enjoyment is triggered in this way because of some individual connections in our brains, some mysterious neurons which make these people called sado-masochists find their delight in the infliction and/or receiving of pain and humiliation (in a sexual context – that proviso is all-important).' Deborah confessed that she could only get turned on by a cane or some other instrument of punishment figuring in the encounter, although outside the bedroom she was dominant. So, she said, 'Stop asking "why?" just lie back and enjoy it (or in my case, bend over and enjoy it)'.

I couldn't help it. Why? Why? Why?

Sensing that her line of thought might provoke scepticism from right-thinking women, she went on to argue against those feminists 'who have bound themselves into a strait-jacket of their own party-line orthodoxy which has become more restrictive than a Victorian whalebone corset . . . are in effect attempting to hold back true liberation, because an admission that women are no longer oppressed would destroy their own *raison d'être*.' I'm no fan of Andrea Dworkin or Catherine MacKinnon but I think Deborah was overstressing her case, unless I was out the day women were finally liberated.

These feminists, so Deborah argued, were envious. 'Trapped in their own drabness, feminists envy those who have the courage to enjoy life.' Deborah shared the belief held by most of the groups I'd come into contact with that people who had unusual sexual interests were likely to be of above average intelligence. Which meant that, over the last few months, I had seen every member of Mensa in the buff.

Deborah's above average intelligence enabled her to hypothesise that having a good sex life (in whatever mode of expression fulfilled one's needs) contributed to the development of a better-balanced person. Therefore, 'if Hitler had had a real woman instead of the dimwitted and avaricious Eva, maybe the Holocaust would not have happened. I am not trivialising the worst horror in the bloodstained history of this world, but I read somewhere that at pre-war parties, Hitler always tried to chat up Jewesses, preferring them to the insipid Aryan blondes. One can imagine how those ladies reacted to the insignificant, ill-educated man. But looking back and saying "if only . . ." is an unproductive exercise.'

If only I hadn't written to Lady O, I thought, unproductively. My IQ would have remained incredibly low and I could have still enjoyed being a drab, envious feminist. But if I was now feeling (erotically) tormented, I could draw some comfort that Deborah, too, was feeling the strain. 'We must still be secretive. Gays came out, but sado-masochism never attained that illusory acceptance . . . We shall never achieve general acceptance because ordinary folk are incapable of understanding the refinement of erotica. It is far too good for them. We are the lucky ones because we have found what turns us on, and contentment in that direction sets us free to pursue other aims.'

Such as writing. The Lady O Society produced its own

book list, and I assumed most of the titles were written by Deborah herself. As one of those 'ordinary folk', I was at a loss as to understanding the refinement of titles like *Residential Course, The Domestic Service Agency* and *The Rent Collector*. In an attempt to prove I wasn't as dumb as somebody like Deborah would think, I took out my notebook and jotted down some titles for erotic fiction to be written at a later date. I came up with *The LEB Power Key, Polyester Blouson* and *The Gherkin Factory*. There, Debs. How's that for erotic refinement?

What of the other Lady Oers? Who were these lucky contented ladies? The contact ads answered my question:

Stefanie: Submissive slut – re-educated former dominant, seeks correspondence and more with males/females of all persuasions. I am tall, long-legged, obedient and eager to be trained in all aspects of slavery.

Rochelle: Submissive blonde petite twenty-three-year-old female wants someone to share my school uniform experiences and fantasies.

Ann: Deeply submissive woman who achieves continual orgasms submitting to be well punished with whip/cane, etc.

Other women sent in letters of support. The Lady O Society was a broad church: Josephine loved being a submissive woman and combining it with her roles as mother, homemaker and career woman. Despite this admirably full timetable, Josephine still found time to worship regularly. What goes on behind closed doors, wondered Josephine, as 'no-one will ever know if any among those neat bottoms kneeling at the communion rail come Sunday carry lines'.

Another letter was a defence of the 'male point of view'. Steffi told all about her and her man. Her punishment from her master took a variety of forms 'from the caning of my bottom and breasts through torturous bondage, inflatable appendages, nipple and clitty clamps, enemas and electrical stimulation. The list goes on and on and there is *always* something new on the horizon being tried out'. I wondered if she'd tried lithium. Steffi ended her letter by saying, 'Stay safe, y'all,' though with electrified clitty clamps, this seemed a little impractical.

Men could be associate members of the society and one letter from a 'gentleman' showed the problems slaves could get into with their Mistresses. 'I think the Lady O Society should campaign for a change in the law to give greater rights to co-habiters . . . I signed my house over to my Mistress and then she threw me out.'

Deborah replied, 'There are plenty of laws to prevent fools and their money from being parted, yet it still happens. And it is certainly not uncommon to hear of subs, male or female, being taken for meal tickets. If you are truly a slave, you should be happy that your Mistress is now much happier, owning property and without you under her feet. Of course you're not. You were playing a different game and you didn't communicate well enough to perceive this.'

Even a drab feminist such as myself could appreciate the beauty of the Lady O Nature Notes which pointed out that it was the time of year when birch-rods were most supple and nettles ('a wonderful instrument of torture') were readily available, though I think I'd already read the same thing in *The Country Diary Of An Edwardian Lady*. But I tarried no longer with The Lady O Society as I had bigger fish to fry . . .

My letterbox had gone quiet. Too quiet. On the rare occasions when the postman rang twice, I would bolt to the door and sniff my post. Nothing. After coming so close, the trail had gone cold. Someone had squawked. The Punctuator had flown the coop.

About a week after my last contact with Enhance, an unobtrusive letter arrived on my doorstep. I had sniffed it as usual and had thrown it to one side. Then it hit me. It was faint, barely registering, little more than a memory but it was there. The vein just below my eyebrow began to throb. That was my second sense talking and I listened. I retrieved the missive from a pile of begging letters and tore it open. A green credit card fell out. But it wasn't Access. Emblazoned across the front and picked out in gilt were the words, 'Communication' and 'Understanding'. Touchy, feely, cary, shary and just a little bit scary – it could only be the work of one person. She was back!

Along with my Enhance membership card (for it was this), Gillian had sent me the new issue of the club magazine, a video list and, to make up for her absence from my letterbox, two letters each containing the same information but a different number of asterisks. Two of these punctuation marks and the first clause of a sentence had been high-lighted but then . . . the high-lighter pen ran out!*! Such calamity had taken its toll on Gillian as she said, 'I must apologise for periodic delays in response to some personal letters during the past year, but I have been in and out of hospital . . .' Of course, the

Erotic Tormental Hospital. Why hadn't I checked there first?

Gillian wrote that I should feel free to enter into correspondence on any matter I so wished, as she had considerable experience of most subjects covered by Enhance and could give me advice about sources and specialist items and practices. 'There is no need for inhibition in correspondence with Gillian,' said Gillian. 'You can be as explicit as you wish and you can expect the reply to be equally uninhibited.' To do so, though, I had to send her twelve stamps or make a £5 donation or send a Stabilo six-pack. My first letter would ask why she had begun to refer to herself in the third person and enquire about the Titan rinse. My second would be to ask why it took twelve stamps to answer the first.

Before I could do that, I had to check out the video list and the magazine. The video list contained all the usual suspects that had been playing at the NFT for years. *Rubber Solution* from Germany featured 'a rubber clad nun who runs a clinic where various treatments are carried out by rubber clad females. Anal, enema, W.S., rubber gear, masks, tubes etc. Very strong!' *El Chalet* from England was made at a Spanish ET hotel. 'Action starts with two naked ladies having a whip fight on the lawn, then moves to dungeon.' There were two films that I hadn't managed to catch in repertory. One was the English *Eels for Pleasure*, which was not, as I originally thought, set in a pie and mash shop. The other was the *German Shit-Lover 5*, a playful pastiche of one of the earlier more difficult works from Fassbinder.

From the magazine, I began to suspect that some Class B psychedelics may have been partly to blame for Gillian's altered state. Where psychiatrists have ruminated for aeons on the origins of sexual paraphilias, Gillian was crystal clear. 'It seems the days are gone by when the playgrounds were filled with pairs of girls with skipping ropes in their mouths as reins, playing "Ponies" or "Chariots", with a friend driving them/holding the reins. And those more private games of "Cowboys and Indians" that introduced many a boy or girl to the exciting sensation of bondage and those of playing "Doctors and Nurses", that taught us in a far more practical way, about the anatomy of the sexes!' I was frightened by the insight. What damage to my psyche had been caused by all those years of KerPlunk-abuse?

This theme was developed further in a piece entitled 'Ride A Cock-Horse' which appeared, I think, in a truncated form in the *British Journal of Psychiatry*. On the subject of horses, the writer wondered if the economic climate had affected little girls having their dream possession, and if so 'whether the sensations of bumping up and down on a saddle and the joy of controlling such a beast, still leads to recreating of these in sexual games later in life?' So buying a child a My Little Pony is no better than buying them nipple clamps. And Thelwell is just a Ladybird edition of de Sade.

I had a horse as a child but aside from a slight bowing of the legs and a thing about Lester Piggott, I had emerged relatively unscathed from this deviance. There were however, according to the piece, others less fortunate who had gone on to develop a taste for riding humans instead of horses. 'The nude mount may be harnessed i.e. halter with bit and reins, hoof-boots and gloves and even a saddle. (Though many will prefer the direct contact between the steed's back and the rider's bare bottom/crotch, as this adds a certain piquancy to the situation, for there can be a certain amount of ooz-ing or even excited spurts as the rider becomes aroused, making for some slip-sliding as the mount is urged to the trot or canter, by switch and spurred boots!)'

The software developed to facilitate this particular sport would have Lucinda Pryor Palmer rolling in her horse box. A 'crupper' was a crotch strap which could hold an anal rod or plug and this was very useful for holding a tail. These harnesses could also incorporate penile/genital restraints and encumbrances. Reins could be attached to nipples and other sensitive parts if they were pierced, if not, clamps offered 'alternative attachment-points'.

For authenticity, it was suggested that these games take place in surroundings similar to a stable, with an out-house serving as a stable box. The ponies should be nude to accentuate their vulnerability while the trainer should be wearing boots with spurs and carrying a whip. 'A leather outfit has its (durable and fearsome) merits but rubber is waterproof and easily cleaned, for unpre-dictable conditions can exist!' Peculiarly, the piece was illustrated with a photograph of Su Pollard atop a man on all fours (both fully dressed) taken at a scene party. The article went on at length. By now I had gotten the gist and with a Hi-de-Hi-Ho Silver, I was away.

Further on, Gillian turned once again to the subject of CP. As per usual, safety was paramount, she felt, in exploring erotic torments, tastelessly using the fate of Joy Gardner to ram home her warning, accompanied by drawings of the 'Home Office Restraints' used in that particular case. Each year, she said, 'over one hundred deaths occur from using partial-suffocation to provide vicarious sensual enhancement. The danger lies in their elated state, the need for oxygen may be overlooked and [lead to] unconsciousness, followed by death . . . [as in the Stephen Milligan case].' If only Milligan had written to Gillian. The orange would have still been in the bowl.

Not that Gillian thought that there was necessarily anything wrong with a little heavy-handedness from the long arm of the law, as the next article featured her experiences of receiving corporal punishment for stealing in Hong Kong. It was an effective deterrent but then two nights in the Kowloon hotel I once stayed in would have worked just as well.

Bondage too came under Gillian's safety conscious scrutiny. In a piece entitled, 'Bondage – The Realities', she warned that masturbatory fantasy could become very dangerous when enacted. Tied up and gagged you could suffer gangrene, incontinence from fear, infection from sex, excessive pain, weals, and on and on. Chastened, I flicked on to a piece on 'knicker-wetting/peeing and/or defecation' and kept on flicking. With friends like Gillian, who needed enemas?

From the photo-spread I flicked to, it was clear that Aunty Josie felt she did. Face down on her flokati, Josie, if it was she, was shown enjoying a situation fit for a princess. The photo-spread was entitled 'Rope and Some Household Bits and Pieces', so I took it that a piping bag and a shower attachment were being used in the procedure. I showed the picture to Ben for a positive ID. He confirmed that it was indeed a piping bag but claimed that Aunty Josie only had lino down.

My membership entitled me to free personal ads so I had a quick look through the lonely hearts column. The ads went along the lines of:

Have gag will travel? Female or females required, must be well qualified in the art of gagging. Applicants will be preferably able to demonstrate an above average working knowledge of the topic and related skills. We are sub/dom male and sub female. (Wigan, Lancs, Anywhere).

I could gag along with the best of them but there was something about that 'Anywhere' which sounded a little bit too desperate.

Now that Josie was safely out of the frame, my reasons for staying with Enhance were diminishing. Although I feared for her sanity at times, Gillian in her numerous contrite articles, seemed fairly aware of the power that her position afforded her. I began to see that her addiction to administration was a form of therapy for her. Hitting the asterisk key stopped her hitting out at the world. As a parting shot, Gillian admitted that she was no longer able to guarantee the three-month cycle of publishing on time. I deduced from this that Gillian was as close to being cured as she would ever be. I closed the casebook, slightly saddened that I would never find out the secret of a Titan rinse.

Chapter 9

PUTTING ON
A LITTLE SHOW

Not surprisingly, my correspondence with Gillian and Deborah did nothing to revive my flagging interest in sex. I was half thinking about giving up totally but this thing had gained its own momentum. At the Safer Planet Sex Ball I had been given a contact address for a swingers' group called the Ring of Confidentes who claimed they stood for celebration sex and fantasy fulfilment. I'd joined and forgotten about it. But along with the last of the letters from Gillian, I received a rather convivial letter from 'PT' at the Ring. One of the main reasons I joined the group was that it didn't cost anything to do so. I was a bit worried that not having a membership fee would encourage the riff-raff element, but then the Party Susan Club hadn't actually been full to the rafters with Lucie Clayton graduates. PT said the reason they didn't charge was because 'we all benefit from widening our circle of like-minded friends'. So far on the swinging scene I hadn't met any friends with minds like mine, but I lived in hope.

The Ring's next get-together, said the letter, was likely to be a small party in London where, if I preferred, I was very welcome just to watch others. 'Let's face it,' he wrote (I don't think that it was sexist of me to assume that PT was a man), 'many of us like being watched anyway!' Furthermore, if the weather improved, then some outdoor amusements were on the cards.

PT expanded on this theme. 'Considerable enjoyment can still be had without necessarily indulging in full physical exchanges. For example, have you ever wanted to watch a couple make love, or [partake in] other intimate acts, whilst you observe either seen or unseen – or put on a little show yourselves? We like to have fun in many different settings, such as car-parks, woods, parties, naturist beaches, saunas and clubs. The only qualities we insist upon are total lack of selfishness/pushiness, an appreciation of eroticism and a sense of humour!' That clinched it. If they wanted a self-effacing woman to laugh at them while they were making out in a Sainsbury's car-park then I was their girl. I could shop during foreplay, come out for the big finish and with my receipt their parking would be free. Which was assuming that when they did it in a car-park they were actually in a car. They couldn't do it in a shopping trolley. Could they?

I was invited to write a brief description of myself detailing my interests and preferences. I included Ben – Dominic now being totally disinterested in pursuing his group-sex fantasy – who, it must be said, has himself known love in an NCP lot. I said I was AC/DC (although PT said this was not necessary, I believe it always gets a warm reception in these circles). Hesitancy was my ace card and I said how we were newcomers to the swinging scene who would like to go further in a non-threatening environment. Though preferably not Surrey Quays Tesco's, as my mother shops there.

A week later, I received a phone call from the organiser, Pete T, an insurance broker from north London. Like many of the males on the swinging scene he sounded middle aged and middle class. We talked for a few minutes about the Safer Planet Sex Ball, where he admitted he'd been active in one of the drive-in cars and had, unfortunately, got his head stuck through the sun roof during the Big O.

Pete then launched into an attack on the swinging scene, saying many groups frowned on you if you didn't discard your clothes on the doorstep and this was not what the Ring of Confidentes was like. 'We have all faced a lifetime of sexual conditioning and there are many people who would like to explore their sexuality in a non-threatening environment,' he said.

I readily agreed. He went on to tell me that the group worked as a forum for ideas. The Ring was about matching up people with similar requirements and at the party I could fill in a questionnaire as to my particular needs. But Pete didn't seem to be able to wait for the questionnaire.

'Any fantasies you and Ben would like to explore?' he asked.

Well, I used to pretend to be Dora from *Follyfoot*. 'A few, yes.'

Pete soon cottoned on to the fact that if he wanted me to talk dirty I was going to need some coaxing. 'Do you enjoy watching guys and girls masturbate?' he asked.

Dora really knew how to wear a cowl neck. 'Er, I suppose so.'

'I'm an exhibitionist! I love people seeing me come,' laughed Pete.

'Ha!' I laughed back.

Pete changed his tack to try and elicit something more from me than a grunt. 'Although we're not into the body-perfect we do like people to be clean, presentable, attractive, to have reasonably looked after their bodies and to be relatively articulate. Have you and Ben gone to seed?'

I didn't know what to say. These things are all relative. Compared to Cindy Crawford, yes. Compared to Peggy Lee, no. Betting that the Ring had more Peggys than Cindys I hazarded a no.

Pete went on. 'There's going to be fifteen couples at the party. You can get a lot of titillation from just groping and fondling. Have you ever had group sex?'

Actually, I've never been able to get more than two people in the back of a Ford Fiesta. 'I've been having a threesome,' I lied. I didn't want the man to think that I was a virgin.

'Oh, well,' jumped in Pete, 'if we have a mutual attraction at the party you can put me down for that one.'

I'd walked right into it.

Pete kindly sent on the questionnaire along with the party invite. The ten questions included: Would you like to watch an (a) man (b) woman masturbate? Would you like to masturbate in front of (a) males (b) females? Would you have a threesome with (a) two males (b) two females? Would you like to go to a sex workshop? Are you prepared to have full-blown intercourse with a fifty-year-old man in white shoes and trousers with an elasticated waistband? At the bottom it said, 'If you've answered no to all the above then you are probably a tabloid journalist and should leave before the fun starts.' I crossed out all our 'Nos' and said maybe to everything. If he took off the shoes maybe it wouldn't be so bad.

A month later, we traipsed across town to a rather dingy-looking house in north-west London. When Ben saw it his spirits dropped and they hadn't been high to start with. 'Great,' he said, 'another evening watching common people take their clothes off.'

I knocked on the door.

'Fifteen minutes and then we're leaving,' he went on. 'I'm not going to (a) masturbate in front of, or (b) be masturbated in front of. If a single drip of bodily fluid lands on my trousers . . .'

The door opened and we were greeted by Pete and his co-organiser, Dave. Both happily single, though I did have the sneaking suspicion that Pete had a wife locked away somewhere. It's a rule of thumb that the invariably male organisers of swingers' groups will invariably be single and invariably insist that everybody else be part of a couple. What do these men think they've got to trade? We were shown into the kitchen where there were six people who seemed to be sharing a bottle of wine between three. Fortunately, we had brought our own reserves and when Pete offered us a glass of Concorde we proffered our two bottles of Chardonnay and asked for one to be opened. Without turning away from the kitchen cabinets, we downed the best part of a bottle.

Looking around, I found, as usual, the talent to be

sadly lacking. Wasn't there one drop dead gorgeous snake-hipped man out there with an overwhelming urge to swing? I had the suspicion that there were quite a few, only they were going to better parties than me.

'See that woman over there?' Ben pointed to a woman dressed in a white fanny pelmet skirt and white fishnet stockings who was sandwiched between two very anaemic-looking blond men on the sofa. 'She'll be the first to unclip her sussies.'

The woman's name was Samantha and although I didn't wish to judge a book by its cover, when that cover said *Razzle*, I had to agree. Samantha was gagging for it. If the clothes one was wearing were a sign of intent, the fact that I was wearing a dress down to my ankles over a roll-on and near-surgical stockings said a loud, 'Go thither'.

Pete made introductions and did his spiel on the group's *raison d'être*. For over a year, around eighty people had used the Ring to make their fantasies come true. Pete was something of an erotomaniac's Jimmy Saville. He seemed genuine enough but I did have a nagging suspicion that the Ring was more about making his own fantasies come true than anybody else's. He did ask us if anyone knew how to operate a video professionally, as two members wanted to make an erotic video of themselves. He reiterated that there was no pressure on anybody to do something they didn't want to.

He left us in the hallway to talk to a couple, Jane and Mark, who seemed out of place on the swinging scene as neither one of them looked as if they were suffering from a vitamin deficiency. From their open-toed sandals, you could tell they espoused the idea of free love but I didn't think they'd find anything at the Ring of

Confidentes which would embody the spirit of '68. The spirit of Dunkirk, maybe. Jane and Mark were into the fetish scene and I soon found out that Jane and I had more in common than a lack of attraction to swingers. At the Safer Planet Sex Ball, she too had been approached by a transvestite in the toilets.

'What did he say to you?' As if I needed to ask.

'Something about me looking saucy and did I want some action.'

Pete came back to shoo us into the living-room to appreciate the buffet he'd laid on. 'Have you eaten yet?' he asked.

He should have said, 'How d'ya like them apples?' as the buffet consisted chiefly of them. Maybe they were Pete's token nod to lewd food. Maybe we were going to have a bra-less bobbing competition. Or maybe, and I think this is more likely, Pete just didn't have a clue. As I ruminated on a Pippin, I watched Samantha squirming on the sofa. If somebody didn't take her brakes off soon, her engine was going to overheat. As Pete passed around the fruit bowl, he introduced us to another couple, Barbara and Richard. She was a tall, blonde school-teacher and he was a less tall, dark-haired, porn-film lighting director. After talking to them for five minutes, it was clear we were kindred spirits. I think if Barbara had been approached by Saucy Mark too, we would have swapped on the spot. They too, were on something of a sexual odyssey. If the right scene were to happen, then maybe they were up for it, but in the meantime they were happy just to laugh at men in their underpants; which is precisely what we spent most of the evening doing.

All of a fluster, Pete broke into our conversation.

'There's some hot action going on in the bedroom!'

I looked around. The sofa was empty. Bar for a wet spot. Obediently, the whole party decamped to the bedroom. Samantha was on the bed with the two men who looked as if they'd been grown in the dark. She'd abandoned the fanny pelmet but the sussies were still in place. All that revving up must have flooded her engine as the sex seemed desperately enervated. She listlessly grasped one bull by the horn whilst lethargically riding bronco atop the other. All that you could see of her steed were his legs sticking out at the bottom.

'Look at his foot,' whispered Ben and I did. It was wrapped in a greying bandage.

Maybe he heard Ben, because a muffled voice came out from between Samantha's knees, 'We're going on strike'. And they were already on a go-slow.

'Oh, no, you're not,' I shouted in encouragement. 'I left my apple to come and watch this.'

It worked. Samantha rolled off and began switching between penises, sucking noisily on each, like a child torn between a Strawberry Mivvi and a Funny Face. A man sidled up to me fondling his crotch. He asked me if I'd ever been to an erotic party before. I said nothing and moved closer to Ben who was still transfixed by the bandage. All around the room people were groping the crotch of the person standing next to them. All except me, Ben, Barbara and Richard. The daisy chain stopped here.

We soon tired of Samantha and friends and returned to the kitchen to finish off our second bottle. Pete reappeared and said, 'Would the ladies like to come and watch me perform?'

Hoping against hope he meant a medley from 'Mack

and Mabel', I said yes. As he went off to warm up, I said to Barbara, 'He did buy the apples. It's the least we can do.'

She didn't look convinced.

I took it upon myself to press-gang the other women present into accompanying us to the second bedroom. I met with some resistance from a very attractive and feisty Australian woman called Paula who only gave in under duress. Shoving her into the bedroom, I could see Ben looking like a rabbit caught in the headlights, silently mouthing, 'Don't leave me here on my own'.

Pete jumped up on the bed and began taking his clothes off. Underneath his trousers he was wearing a red and none too masculine posing pouch. Jane beat a hasty retreat, her sandals barely touching the Axminster. I could hear her in the hall saying to Ben, 'I am not watching a man do that in women's underwear'.

Meanwhile, back in the bedroom, Pete's hot love action was going down a storm. 'Get it off,' we roared.

Pete took it off and bounced up and down. Oh, how we applauded.

'It's lovely,' I said. 'But it's not hard.'

Pete bounced some more. 'It gets more difficult when you're the wrong side of forty.'

Wrong side of forty? He looked like a man who could remember where he was the day Archduke Ferdinand was shot. To encourage his endeavours, I let him squeeze my breasts. Or rather the padding in my bra. Feeling an inch of nylon polyamide webbing seemed to do the job and his manliness rose until we were eye to eye. And what a huge eye Pete had. 'What a huge eye you've got,' I said and suddenly it was winking at the floor again.

To rectify the situation, Pete moved his attentions to Paula, who, despite her initial reluctance, was now finding comfort in another woman's bosom. Or padding as the case may be. Faced with old cyclops bearing down on them they broke away from their embrace and gave Pete an encouraging rub of the calf muscles. Bouncey bouncey went Pete.

It was odd that while Barbara and I were fighting to get out of the bedroom, men were fighting to get in. They seemed none too keen on having their women monopolised by one man's big business. The bedroom was quite small, barely enough room for one fully engorged member, and very soon there were four or five of them flying about. You had to duck to avoid the drips.

Having been to a couple of swingers parties by now, I was beginning to develop a theory about what happens. It's not sexual excitement, more mass hysteria. The only thing I can compare it to is a demonstration that turns nasty. One minute you're walking along minding your own business and the next you're spitting at the police and calling them pigs. It's mob rule. One just gets caught up in the moment. Then again, maybe it's like watching the Home Shopping Channel. You may be laughing yourself stupid but all of a sudden, you're on the phone ordering yourself a housecoat with matching *diamanté* earrings. You know damn right it's tacky, but you do it all the same.

Having lost the spotlight, Pete had slouched off into the other bedroom. I found Ben in the kitchen drinking Concorde straight from the bottle.

'Paula's got really big feet,' he said. 'I've been wearing her shoes.'

Before I had a chance to ask why, Pete popped in in his pouch and said, 'Come and see what Dave is doing. He's got a whopper.'

I took Ben with me for protection, although by this point he was listing at an alarming angle.

In bedroom one, a man was fucking his girlfriend on the bed. He was naked, bar for his shirt, so I guess he had a problem with underarm swoop. Next to them, Dave was being sucked off by, you've guessed it, Samantha.

'Honestly,' said Ben. 'Give that woman six inches and she'll take a mile.'

It was pretty hard to tell if Dave had a whopper or not, as Samantha seemed most reluctant to let any of it out of her mouth. I felt I had to show some willing and participate a bit. So as a tribute to Party Susan's Wiggy, I went over to Dave and smacked him on the bottom. Hard. He jerked forward in surprise and Samantha bit down to save her windpipe.

Ben said, 'I need an apple,' and went back into the living-room.

I hit Dave a few more times, laughed a castrator's laugh and left to see what else was happening.

I was stopped in the hall by the crotch rubber. He was now only wearing a pair of very large and unattractive Y-fronts. Actually, quite a few of the men there were wearing similar knickers, so maybe they were the regulation Ring drawers. Pushing past him I said, 'Either take them off or put your clothes back on. You look revolting'.

The orgy in bedroom two had grown since I last looked. Surprisingly, Richard was in the middle, although he defended himself by saying that he still had his trousers on. Barbara barged in to give him what for, but quickly ended up on the bed snogging him. As soon as she lay down next to him, another man swooped in, pulled up her dress and began interfering with her gusset.

'I'm not stoned enough for this,' she said, getting off the bed and rearranging herself.

I felt something rubbing up against my leg. The crotch rubber had dropped his skids. Having regularly experienced rush hour on the tube, the act held no novelty value, so I went off to see how Ben was enjoying his apple.

Back in the living-room, I had the shock of my life. Ben had a stick of celery in one hand and Paula's labia in the other. He wasn't actually eating the celery as he was too busy biting her neck. I think Ben would have gone for the housecoat, the earrings and the matching tiara set. As Paula went for his flies, I stepped in and led him away. His boyfriend would thank me for it later.

Pete reappeared and asked Barbara and me to accompany him into the bathroom to watch him finish his big number. I propped Ben up outside the door and told him to stay there. Pete stood in the bath with one foot on the sink and started to masturbate. Barbara had to stick her head out of the door to laugh.

'For God's sake sing something!' she shouted to Ben.

Pete reached his crescendo accompanied by a lovely a cappella version of 'Oh, Sweet Mystery of Life, At Last I've Found You' being sung through the keyhole.

Not waiting around to savour Pete's afterglow, I came out of the bathroom. Ben was nowhere to be seen. I rushed into bedroom number two. He was on the bed with Paula taking off his clothes. Thinking fast, I offered myself up in sacrifice. Squeezing myself in between them, Paula turned her attention to my thighs.

'Do yourself up,' I hissed at Ben as Paula's hand

edged towards my knicker elastic. Ben buttoned up and left the room. After a discreet interval I followed him. He was in the kitchen talking to Pete and Barbara. Pete asked him, 'Are you going to give the ladies a treat and take off your clothes?'

Barbara was laughing. 'Ben, you couldn't possibly be wearing any more clothes than you are.'

It was true. Although I was fighting for his dignity, it would have taken Paula a good ten minutes to get him anywhere near naked.

'I took my balaclava off when I came in,' said Ben indignantly, rummaging around for more drink.

It was about twelve o'clock when everyone started to disappear. We said goodbye to Barbara and Richard. In the kitchen, I bumped into the man who had kept his shirt on while seeing to his girlfriend.

'Did you come?' I asked, trying to make conversation.

'No.'

'Why not?'

'I couldn't do that in front of a woman,' he replied.

'What, you can't come in front of a woman?' I asked, incredulously.

'Oh, I thought you said, "Did you fart?"'

I thought it was time to take Ben home. We went to say goodbye to Dave. He was sitting on the bed in bedroom one looking sulky. He pulled me down by his side and said there had been a complaint about me. Some man had moaned that I kept hitting him.

I twigged on, 'It was you, Dave, wasn't it?'

He changed the subject. 'You've got a lovely arse,' he said. 'Why have you kept your clothes on all night?'

Feeling guilty for nearly losing him his wedding tackle

and not wanting to be upstaged by Ben, I walked over to the corner of the room, pulled down my tights, struggled womanfully with my roll-on, bent over and gave him a show. This was cut short when I lost my balance, toppled over and hit my head on a wardrobe door. Time to go.

Paula said goodbye at the door. 'Look after him, he's very vulnerable.'

Ben gave her a cheesy grin.

Outside, I heard something clanking in Ben's bag.

'I've stolen two bottles of wine,' he said

'Take them back,' I ordered. 'Well . . . take one back.'

Still infused with eroticism, we offered the cab driver a blow job in lieu of the fare. He gave me a kiss and took my £20.

Chapter 10

DINNER
À
DOUZE

The next day, rising late from my revelries, I threw on the same dress I'd been wearing the night before, as I was on my way to my friend's wedding. At the reception, Dominic took me to one side to whisper a very important sweet nothing. It was a marriage proposal, to which I said yes. Dominic said that he thought he should get in quick as it appeared that I had another serious admirer.

'What makes you think that?' I asked, slightly worried about what he thought he knew.

'The dried cum down the back of your dress kind of gives it away,' he said, matter of factly.

Hastily retiring to the powder room, and in the process missing The Bride's First Dance followed shortly after by The Bride's First Row, I found that one of the Confidentes had indeed popped his cork down the back of my dress. You'd think a marriage proposal and the humiliation of parading a jism-stained frock in front of my friend's grandparents would have been enough to stop my sexual investigation dead in its tracks. But in a funny way I'd enjoyed the Ring party, even though I'd abandoned any thoughts that I'd find something out there that would really excite me. Besides, I still had to work.

To this end, I joined Forum, which was something of a Swingers' Guild. Originally associated with *Forum* magazine, the organisation branched off in 1980. Cerig, Forum's national organiser, sent me its information pack. It introduced itself thus: 'Forum groups had been in existence for nearly as long as *Forum* magazine and over the years they'd emerged from being discussion groups to actually participating in recreational sex. Nowadays, Forum groups are accepted as serious contributors to the International Alternative Lifestyle movement.'

Forum has a 'safe sex' code and categorises each swingers' group according to their preferred level of engagement. 'D' for discussions; social gatherings but no sex. 'N' for non ultimate; social nakedness and touching/caressing, but sex only with one's regular partner. 'C' for condom; recreational sex permitted but only when using a condom. 'R' for restricted; this code applies to small intimate groups where all are happy with each other's lifestyle. Condoms are not deemed necessary but new members may have to abide by code 'C' for an initial period. Some groups may favour more than one category for different occasions.

I was depressed by the wilful stupidity displayed. I wanted to track down an R group and ask them just how they check out people's lifestyles. Can you be a member of more than one R group? Just how many people are you allowed to swing with before your lifestyle is deemed unacceptable? And what does wearing a condom for the first few times prove? Still, there was a token commitment to safer sex, all Forum members had to abide by the SASH rule – Swing And Stay Healthy. Abiding by my own admittedly less punchy rule, IWSWMWWWS (I Won't Sleep With Men Who Wear White Shoes), I sent off the £30 membership fee.

Scanning through the club listings, I came across a group which sounded right up my street called 'One Step At A Time'. This was a 'Swingers for Beginners' group which had been formed especially for hesitant couples who wanted to swing but didn't want to be pushed. The group was committed to socialising with a 'completely frank exchange of ideas'. I put pen to paper immediately. There were a lot of things about swingers that I wanted to be completely frank about. Not least their soft furnishings.

   I got a bit carried away with myself writing the letter. I'd just seen *Jules et Jim* and, fancying myself as the Hackney Jeanne Moreau, said once again that Ben and I had until recently been in a threesome with another man. Having enjoyed the experience we were now hoping to go further afield – but hesitantly.

   A couple of days later the phone rang early in the morning. Nursing a terrific hangover, I answered it expecting it to be a complaint about my behaviour the night before, as it so often is. But it was Richard, One Step At A Time's top step. He was calling to invite me to a party, but I couldn't make the date.

   'Maybe the next one,' I said. 'How often do you have them?'

'Well, the last one was a year ago.'

They certainly were hesitant.

Richard explained that the club had been on its last legs but had suddenly had a new wave of interest. Which I think probably meant that I'd been stupid enough to write.

'What are you into?' he asked.

'Ooh, all sorts . . .' I still couldn't get the hang of talking dirty on the phone.

He waited for me to elaborate, which didn't happen, then asked, 'So why did the threesome stop? What happened to your other man?'

In a fit of passion, I tossed back my red hair and drove our car over Lambeth Bridge. I survived the fall and went on to become a great character actress while he lies still in a watery grave. 'He moved.'

'So would you like another man to take his place?'

If this was One Step At A Time, I would hate to see Jumping Straight In With Both Feet. 'Erm . . .'

'Maybe it's too early in the morning for you to talk about things like this?'

Too early in my hangover at least. Richard left it there and promised to write.

His letter arrived a few days later. In it, Richard said another reason for the group being a bit moribund of late was 'because Alison [his partner] has been going through a rather introspective phase herself, from which we both hope she will emerge in due course . . .' For 'introspective phase' should I read 'nervous breakdown'? Richard wasn't about to let his partner's indisposition hold him back as he finished the letter by saying, 'And if you might be contemplating the recruitment of a second male to join you for an occasional saucy evening, I'd love to meet up to see if we hit it off. Alison doesn't wish to see me deprived of the odd injection of excitement!' Testament, indeed, to the powers of Prozac.

Deciding that 'hesitant swinger' was an oxymoron, I gave the One Step At A Time club the bum's rush. In the same post as Richard's letter came my Forum membership. Attached to it was a discreet lapel badge depicting a silver dove on black enamel which one could wear to identify oneself as a Forum member or, perhaps, a peacenik. Along with the lapel badge you could also send off for the car windscreen version which fits inside a tax-disc holder. Personally, I think the 'Drive Slowly: Adult Baby On Board' stickers are identification enough.

They had also included, at my request, an information leaflet on starting up your own group. This noted that many Forum groups have a couples-only rule – 'unfair perhaps but then the Forum scene is primarily for people who have come to terms with their sexuality and lead well-adjusted sex lives. This precludes men who find it difficult to form satisfactory relationships with women . . .' Let's review that last point: Moira, the wife of Party Susan's Adam, had run off, Confidente Pete seemed to have mislaid his wife and Richard's partner was suffering from 'introspection'. Were they men who could form satisfactory relationships with women?

According to Forum they were. Forum believed that maladjusted men were in the minority on the swinging scene. The leaflet said that with the growth of threesomes (two men and a woman) added to the fact that women could far surpass men in sexual performance and may, therefore, want multiple partners, many groups were allowing single men in.

Forum members, it said, tended to be above average in status (I think the expression is 'all fur coat and no knickers') and, as a consequence, tried to avoid scandal. Some of the groups did indeed try to present themselves as being upmarket in their ads. For example, Sensual Encounters was 'an established but loose organisation of liberated, cultured people who prefer to meet in small encounter groups . . . organiser is a skilled masseur'. Or, there was Wiltshire Cottage, a snappy title for a group that was highly selective and welcomed non-promiscuous, friendly people with social skills, high libido and a sense of humour.

If hosting a party, you were advised not to get anxious about the sex side of your group but instead enjoy the pleasant social atmosphere, interesting conversation and good company and to let the 'fucking be incidental, *not* the essential part of your group's activity. Everyone knows our interest is in sex and while many members enjoy group sex, some are held back . . . so give them dim lights, soft music, warmth, erotic videos and magazines, undressing games and massage.'

Other tips to help a group go with a swing were to hold discussion meetings, have outside speakers come and talk, or hire a sauna for the night. Apparently, successful groups can grow quickly and reach a hundred members or more. Often they split into smaller groups and the commonest size is twelve to thirty members who usually belong to more than one group.

I also received a few back issues of the *Forum* newsletter. February's made me worry as it was about journalists. As the *News of the World* had just run a swinging exposé, the society wanted to help prevent couples having their private affairs laid bare for everyone to read 'by reporters whose sole aim is to provide titillating and mostly untrue copy for all those who get turned on by reading about it, would love to get involved themselves but are such hypocrites that if their neighbours were caught would instantly condemn them'. As much as I disapproved of the *News of the World*, you had to hand it to their journalists: they were better writers than me if they could provide titillating copy about the swinging scene.

The newsletter also gave advice on weeding out journalists. Beware, it said, anybody appearing to ask too many questions or seeming reluctant to get involved and always demand an undraped photo in your correspondence. This made me instantly suspicious of the man in a vest, posing with his Alsatian in front of his Everest patio doors in one of the photos I'd received from the Party Susan club. He had *Guardian* Women's Page written all over him.

With this warning in mind, I scanned through the Forum contact ads. All the usual suspects were present and correct. All the men were professionals, slim and massively endowed which translates as twenty-three stone, works in Bejams and has less of an endowment than the Mirror Group Pensioners. One such perfect specimen was seeking anything on 'masturbation – books, mags, videos, correspondence, perhaps meet females for group masturbation' but for some reason the idea of circle jerking with a needle-dicked lard-arse didn't appeal. Maybe it was the cold hands.

Despite my reservations, three adverts fired my imagination, although two of them had nothing to do with swinging. The first I wrote to was called 'The Other Pony Club', and, thanks to Gillian from Enhance, I was up to

speed with SM pony activities. And with Ben taking the
bit (not that he knew it) I would get to play Dora from
Follyfoot after all. The second advert read: 'Tantric-
initiated exponent Raja yoga, Catholic priest and
alchemist priestess-of-Isis tutors singles, couples, groups,
in communications, self-discipline and correction'. I
wrote to this one because I didn't have the faintest idea
what was on offer.

The third, Ben picked out. He said that if we had to
go swinging again we were going to go upmarket to do
it. 'Erotic Eats' sounded just the job. 'A group run by a
very charismatic couple who are superb hosts and
gourmet cooks. They hold dinner parties for up to
twelve with the finest wine and champagne. Guests are
encouraged to dress provocatively. If you enjoy good
food, conviviality and sensual pleasures write today.'

So I did and I soon received an invitation to dinner.
Erotic Eats was based in north London and in their
mailout, they promised fine wines and a five-course
meal, followed by the chance to do a little bit of light fingering. After the spread laid on by the Ring of
Confidentes so totally failed to satiate the Epicure in
me, I thought, if I must have my breasts squeezed, wasn't
it better to have them squeezed over a lobster mornay?

Leaving a Vesta curry on the kitchen table for Dominic,
Ben and I went off to Erotic Eats. Standing over the road
from the house where dinner was to be served we
watched two of the guests going in. They looked to be of
an age where dinner might have to go through the
blender before they could eat it. It was quite dispiriting.
Did nobody under a pensionable age want to swing?

'I don't want to go in,' said Ben, whose relationship
had broken down in the afternoon after a sustained

bout of crockery throwing. Ben blamed the split on the stress of accompanying me on my forays, but I'm sure it was just the fact that his boyfriend had finally caught him not holding his stomach in.

'Well you can't eat at home. You haven't got any plates left,' I reasoned.

'I got out of the Oedipal stage at six,' he said sulkily, pointing to Mrs Swinger.

We were greeted at the door by the hosts, Peter and Sue. Peter seemed a good twenty years older than his partner and, again, I wondered why some men feel the need to push their luck. The house was filled with antiques and not all of them were sitting down to dinner. We were shown to the top floor of their house and given a glass of champagne to break the ice. Feeling frosty, I had several more while nobody was looking.

We were introduced to the couple who arrived just before us – Jill and Gerald. They were swinging veterans who'd been exposed by the *News of the World* more times than Maria Whittaker's breasts. They had met at the first Sex Maniac's Ball. They were unsure just how long ago that was, but I would've taken a guess and said that the theme must have been Fanny by Gaslight. Gerald asked me what I had liked about the Planet Sex Ball. Foolishly, I said that one of the best things about it was that there were so many old people there, meaning I admired their spirit. But Gerald immediately took me for a gerontophile and as a chaser for the post-prandials urged Jill to tell us about her encounter with the real oldest swinger in town.

'He was eighty-seven and had been swinging for over sixty years,' said Jill delightedly. 'He was fabulous at oral sex.'

'Presumably because he took his teeth out,' I said, agog.

'No they were in and I don't think they were false. I didn't feel them nip independently.'

A few of the other couples arrived. The most notable were Neil and Eva, mainly because Eva's breasts arrived a good two minutes before she did. Her cup ranneth over and she was obviously unable to locate the stop-cock. She was five feet tall with around two foot of curly blonde acrylic hair which sat on her head looking as if it had escaped from a knitting bag. There must be some correlation between swinging and follicle damage, I thought, remembering the similarly afflicted Wiggy. She was well matched in Neil. He was a Terry Thomas look-alike, wearing, and I still find it hard to believe that he was, a tie in the shape of a penis. Ben choked on his nuts when Neil shot me a look which suggested he'd like me to do the same on his.

Dinner was served in the basement. As I made my way down the stairs, I pleaded with God to be merciful and spare me the trial of being placed next to Neil. But God was obviously in an Old Testament kind of a mood because there were only two seats spare and the boy–girl arrangement meant that I would be passing the port to Neil. Ben didn't fare any better, as Jill made it quite clear that she would be passing something on to him. On the wall in the living-room, I had noticed a framed clipping from the *News of the World* featuring Gerald and Jill. I asked them if they'd minded.

'Well, Jill was annoyed that she was described as my secretary-cum-mistress,' said Gerald.

'The only thing right in that statement is the cum!' screamed Jill, bringing her hand down hard on the table and making the cutlery rattle. Ben looked as if he was going to cry.

There were twelve of us around the table. Opposite me sat Pam and Helmut and next to them, Martin and Nina. Pam informed us that she had been with Helmut for twenty-seven years.

'That's nearly as long as I've been alive!' said Ben as his opening gambit, showing why he doesn't get invited out to dinner that often.

The first course was avocado and King Prawns. It was a toss up which was harder to deal with – Neil or the prawns. I just couldn't bring myself to break their heads off so I gave them to Ben who was still in a destructive mood. Neil's ardour was harder to dismantle. His big joke was mimicking an erection with his tie, and if he did it once he did it twenty times.

As Eva was busy navigating her breasts to get to her plate, she was unable to give Neil the attention he so obviously craved. Out of pity, I asked him what he did for a living.

'I'm a vet,' he said, unaware that his tie was now making love to his avocado.

I looked at his hands. They looked as if they'd be more than comfortable lodged in a cow's rectum.

'And you?' I said to Eva, watching a prawn make its way up through the hills.

'I look after Neil!' she squeaked.

And the twins, I thought, looking at her cleavage. Eva told me she was from Germany and her teeth told me they were from a glass by the side of her bed.

The main course (duck in plum sauce) arrived, and the talk around the table turned to yachts. Monied and middle class, most of the couples present seemed to have one.

'My yacht in Sydney sleeps twelve,' said Martin.

'My mum's caravan is an eight berth,' said Ben, tucking into his duck with his butter knife.

I dislodged Neil's hand from between my thighs and attempted to save Ben from making a complete fool of himself by blundering on about how the cooker pulls down and turns into a couchette for three. I brought the subject back to Australia, intending to rhapsodize about the wonderful skies and landscapes.

'The colours there are so . . .'

'You mean the Aborigines. Ugh!' interrupted Martin.

Although everybody laughed at his mistake, it was clear that most of the people around the table were right behind him. The talk turned to Coolies and how they simply had to use an electric cattle prod on some of their Asian servants to get them to do any work. The assault on my political sensibilities knocked me off guard for a moment, allowing Neil to renew his attack on my crotch. I hoped for his patients' sakes that he was gentler when spaying. Under the tablecloth, Sue had forgone her duck in favour of Gerald's pork. Seeing that her partner was otherwise occupied, Jill (who had undone her blouse during *hors-d'œuvres*) turned her chair to face Ben, took off her knickers, hooked one of her legs over the arm of her chair and threw him a spread. Women have given birth showing less. Ben was having none of it.

Turning his back on her, he hissed at me, 'I'm sorry, but I can't sleep with a woman with a worse perm than my mother.'

Gerald had warned earlier that dessert would be served horizontally. Thankfully, the strawberries and marscapone arrived upright. Eva tucked in.

'I can't believe it's not cream!' she squealed as if she was auditioning for a commercial.

To signify her delight, she unleashed her bosoms. As they flew across the table towards the floral centrepiece the theme tune to *The Dambusters* came into my head. Neil tried to corral them with one hand while taking his trousers off with the other. It wasn't a pretty sight. Neil was an animal lover. I knew this because, aside from being a vet, he was wearing leopard-skin print underpants. When Eva's breasts had settled down to their lowest level, she put her hand into his pants and fished out his penis. Although I was mildly disappointed that it didn't look like a tie, the shock was enough for me to drop one of my strawberries under the table. I left it there for Sue.

Terry tried ministering to Eva's ample frontage. Have you ever seen a mouth trying to find purchase on a football? Without a flip-top head, Terry didn't have a chance. Neil had obviously never managed it either as he went from woman to woman around the table and oozed into their ears, 'Can I suck your tits?' Silken-tongued charmer though he was, to a woman we said no. But he grabbed hold of Pam's anyway. Her face was a picture. That one by Munch.

I needed some cigarettes and, as Jill was still holding her options open, Ben was only too happy to oblige and go out and get some. Once he left, Pam's husband Helmut came and sat down beside me. He was Austrian and keen to give me a Viennese whirl. Before I could say Kurt Waldheim, he had his tongue down my throat and his hand up my dress. Seeing that Ben's seat was free, Eva hoisted herself up off the table and came and took his place. Helmut was transfixed and the Anschluss happened quickly and painlessly. Having annexed Austria, it was clear that Eva saw me in the middle as a potential Czechoslovakia.

Eva undid the front of my dress, her bullet-like nipples grazing my face. 'Do you mind a woman doing this to you?' she purred, scooping my breasts out of my bra. I probably wouldn't, I thought – if she had her own teeth and hair.

Helmut and Eva grabbed a nipple apiece and tugged away like billy-o. Worryingly, Neil had disappeared under the table. For a brief second, I caught sight of him by Eva's beaver and then he was gone again. He wasn't looking for Sue. She was back on her chair and parking a hand in Jill's love drive. On the other side of the table, Pam was squeamishly doing the same to Nina.

'I'm sorry, I just can't do that,' Pam said, essaying a three-point turn.

I felt Neil's head battering at my knees. If I didn't do something the head would soon engage. I was distracted by Eva who was licking my nipples.

'It's like Christmas!' she squeaked.

'Without snow,' I mumbled back into her hairpiece.

I felt trapped. The invasion was coming from all angles. A few smacks to the head had briefly stunned Neil but I knew he would be back. I had to pull out the big gun.

'Ben has got the biggest penis you have ever seen,' I said, lying through my teeth. 'Get him to get it out when he comes back.'

It worked. The attention was deflected from me and I rearranged my foundations. The crowd sat back and waited for Ben's return.

'Get 'em off!' they roared when he walked through the door. Ben looked mortified when I told him what I had said.

'Get your top off,' screamed Jill. It was a double drive.

Ben took off his cardigan and said, 'That's as far as it goes. I need to be wooed.'

On that point he was not to be moved. As some of the blood slowly drained back into my nipples, Martin came over and asked to have sex with me. I could have just about done it for a cruise on his yacht but I lied and said I had my period.

'How frustrating for you,' he said, genuinely feeling sorry for me. 'At the last party we ended up upstairs and one woman had nine orgasms.'

There was no going upstairs that evening. Swinging with the over-fifties does have its advantages. By eleven-thirty they'd started to flag. By twelve they were thinking about their Horlicks. We said our goodbyes and left.

Outside Ben turned to me and said, as he always did, 'Never again.'

And this time, I agreed with him. I had to face it, the swinging scene was never going to do anything for us.

'I wish you'd told me earlier that we wouldn't be going back,' said Ben. 'I would have stolen a couple of plates.'

Chapter 11

AWAY WITH
THE FAIRIES

Dr Colin Hamer's reply was well timed, arriving as it did during a particularly lamentable bathtime rendition of 'Calling Occupants of Interplanetary Craft'. Dr Colin was the face behind the Forum advert, 'Tantric-initiated exponent Raja yoga, Catholic priest and alchemist priestess-of-Isis tutors singles, couples, groups in communications, self-discipline and correction'.

The dirty dinner-party had brought me down again, but Dr Colin must have sensed my spiritual disquiet across the psychic airwaves because his letter fairly dripped with healing. He offered guidance and said that any time I needed his help, I just had to drop him a line. Actually, I would have to drop him two lines as he informed me that all official correspondence should be addressed to: His Benevolence, The Extra-Revd Dr Colin James Hamer DCH, MRP, STL, PhD, AF Phys. (ITEC) Preliminary LibrArian To The Neith Network, The

Rainbow Programme, Creativity House. What a carrier-bag full of credentials His Benevolence possessed! It took me a few minutes to work out that DCH stood for Director of Creativity House and MRP for Master of the Rainbow Programme. STL had me stumped but I'd hazard a guess now at Star Trek Lover. For Dr Colin's philosophy was not affected by the earth's gravitational pull.

The capital A in LibrArian tipped me off to Dr Colin's specialness as did the fact that he habitually missed out the O in G-d. Such a unique approach to grammar could mean only one of two things. Either the Extra-Revd was a true visionary or his typing was being done by The Punctuator. I plumped for visionary because, on the merest of details sent, The Master had divined that Ben was about to complete his first Saturn return within the next year. This alarmed Ben. What if, like Dr Colin, he asked, he was unable to make it all the way back? Immediate comfort was brought when The Director confessed to having just emerged from his second splashdown. As he signed off with 'fun, peace, sharing and zest', I took it that the landing had been a happy one.

Along with his letter, Dr Colin had sent The Neith Network reference list, a videotape and a selection of his papers. The reference list was invaluable. It detailed hundreds of books that promised to answer all those questions you never thought were worth asking on subjects ranging from flying saucers, colour healing, sex and King Arthur to something called morphogenetic resonance pulsation and rhythm vibration medicine. The videotape proved to be as eclectic, featuring, as it did, documentaries on spaceships, Tantric sex, the Amazon and Noah's Ark. The videotape reminded me

of one of those 'What do these four totally unrelated pictures have in common?' type puzzles. The only answer I
could come up with was – the mind of Dr Colin Hamer.

That mind was well displayed in the selection of
papers sent. Said one, 'Locations in Kashmir or elsewhere traditionally designated as "resting-places" of
Jesus may not be tombs but places where his inter-
continental spacecraft touched down. The holy house of
Loreto and the scallop-shells associated both with Venus
and St James of Compostela may also relate to landings
or splashdowns by space capsules.'

The one pressing question left unanswered by Dr
Colin in his selected thoughts was what on earth did
The Preliminary LibrArian have to offer a bunch of
swingers? Could it have been to do with the fact that Dr
Colin believed himself to be a catalytic converter?
'Assisted by Anubis, Maat, Neith, Ptah and other
Angelicals, Colin Hamer functions as a catalytic converter. His gift is that of empowering and enabling
others more clearly to discern how best to effect the
needed transition from a depressing – because of a dis-
ordered situation of frustration and seeming sterility –
to an authenticity chaotic and therefore fertile state of
higher-octave creativity, where each person's life can
grow and flourish more abundantly.'

So there you have it. I felt that Dr Colin had reached
such an exalted state of divinity that the gulf between
our respective understandings would prohibit meaning-
ful intercourse, social or otherwise. But he did give me
an idea. In my search for sexual enlightenment I would
temporarily eschew the corporeal for the ethereal. To
this end, I booked myself a place on a workshop run by
a body called The Serpent Institute. This workshop,

'Wild Woman and Wild Man Meets the Goddess' promised to be a way to explore erotic energy through Goddess spirituality. Which was how, a few days later, I came to be huddled in the corner of a room in a Covent Garden alternative therapy centre, watching in horror as a growling man on all fours tried to eat my shoe.

Wild Women everywhere came out from under their kaftans following the emergence of 'Wild Men' as chronicled by Robert Bly in his book *Iron John*. These Iron Janes were setting out to release feminine sexual energy. This energy, they believed, was once seen as one of the most powerful forces in the universe until it was turned into something evil by men keen to suppress the 'Wild Woman' myth and exert their control over the world. In a bid to reverse this trend, The Serpent Institute had dedicated itself to Goddess Spirituality, focusing on energies, nature, the eco-system, rituals and meditation.

I entered the room where my induction into wild womanism was to take place. I looked around. There were eleven women and two men sitting in a circle. I grabbed myself a scatter cushion, joined them and adopted a serene posture. Being a woman who thought the Lotus position was sticking her legs out of the window of an Esprit, this wasn't easy. Shifting from buttock to buttock, I tuned in to our workshop facilitator, Jocelyn.

The initiation ceremony had begun. Jocelyn explained the need to create a sacred space and evoke the Goddess. This ceremony was intended to separate us from everyday life and allow us space to let go. We were about to be brought into wildness. Inside our ring was a smaller circle made up of paintings of wild women and men. And inside that circle were representations of: emotion – water; the body – stone and crystal; intellect – an incense stick; intuition – a red candle. There was also a wooden snake representing the serpent (female sexual energy) and a sculpture of the eight-thousand-year-old goddess Cybele giving birth.

To reconnect with our true selves we first had to talk about how we felt about our forenames. It transpired that many of the people there felt constrained by the identities that their names constructed for them. To escape from this identity we were given the option to pick a totally new moniker. When one man declared that from henceforth he wanted to be known as 'Og', I knew that the gloves were off. I mumbled something like 'Even a goddess needs to tinkle' and escaped to the toilet for a quick carton of cigarettes. On my return, the stone from the inner circle was being passed around the outer circle. It reminded me of the Orgasmatron scene in Woody Allen's *Sleeper*. No orgasm, though.

Having fondled the rock, we broke into three groups to discuss firstly what wildness meant to us and then, to my absolute horror, to act it out. I was reluctant to recreate my conception of wildness which, going by the average Friday night, required the aid of a wine bar, a set of tattoos and the attentions of a short-order chef named Nikos. Luckily, I had chosen the least demonstrative group who took my lead and decided that doing nothing and looking embarrassed was quite wild enough, thank you.

The rest were far less reticent. Five women aged between twenty-five and fifty roared like animals and threw themselves all over the floor. We, the 'Quietly Wild' women, adopted a David Attenborough-like calm and ducked whenever a paw swiped our way. It got quite ferocious at times. When one of the men pretended to shoot one of the 'animals', I did have the sneaking suspicion he was working through his own agenda.

The other group mimed wild. To an accompaniment of drumming on the floor and chants of 'Om', they acted out scenes of, among other things, rutting and rebirthing. For a moment my cynicism departed and I was transported. There was definitely something in the beat. Feelings of embarrassment and envy mixed as I watched the apparent freedom of the other women. However, my sense of being lost in the rutting and rhythm quickly departed at the thought of being dragged up to rebirth myself.

Fortunately, no-one did. We moved on to another discussion on the meaning of wildness. I wanted to say, for the £40 the workshop cost, I could suggest quite a few ways to go wild. But I kept quiet and picked at the fluff on my gypsy skirt. The others came up with words like intuition, instinct, abandonment (in both senses), rutting, letting go, being true to yourself and not fitting in with other people. Some felt we were getting off the issue of wildness by talking about it. I, on the other hand, was only too happy to stay with the theory rather than the practice.

We were soon on the move again, this time mental travel. We had to relax as Jocelyn told us a modernised version of the Greek myth of Ariadne. The purpose was to guide us into the labyrinth. Ariadne was a high priestess who was abandoned by her human lover on the island of Naxos. Having myself been dumped by an old boyfriend on a Go-Greek package tour, I felt I was Ariadne's sister in suffering. Affiliated to this lovelorn woman, I let her lead me into a cave where I was meant to tell someone close to me things I had never been able to say. Deep in the myth, I found myself thinking morbid, painful thoughts. Lulled by Jocelyn's voice this was powerful but dangerous stuff. I felt uncomfortable with the images that were summoned up from my unconsciousness.

Ariadne couldn't wait for me to sort out my mixed-up emotions. She was back on the ferry and island hopping, off to celebrate her marriage to the god, Dionysus. This was meant to symbolise our letting go and moving into wildness. We were asked to imagine sexual wildness with a partner. Would you believe I missed the best bit. Summoning up the ouzo-laced memory of my Go-Greek idyll (pre-dump) proved too great an exertion and I drifted off to sleep. Although, apparently, I was wonderful.

Lunch finally arrived. In keeping with the mythic tone I had a Mars Bar. It stuck in my throat as I cried down the pay phone to Ben. Originally, he was meant to be experiencing the Goddess with me but had cried off to soak his living-room nets instead.

Post lunch, back in the labyrinth, we danced to the syncopated rhythm of Janna Runnels' 'Eye of the Womb'. This primeval drumming soon had everybody leaping around like Isadora Duncan on Ecstasy. Everybody, that is, except me. Goddess knows, I tried. I collapsed on the floor in silent anguish. It was at this point that the howling 'dog' chowed down on my footwear. Had they been a good pair, I would have slapped him, but I contented myself with the idea that I may have trodden in something on the way in.

The other wild man had taken a shine to one of the

women. I realised that one of the main reasons for my discomfort throughout the day was the presence of the men in the group. I distrusted their motives. Call me without charity, but I wouldn't trust a man who wanted to go on one of these courses. His 'Wild Man' is like all men's – it just wants to cop off.

My suspicion of the men then held me back from partaking in a blindfolded trust game. I wasn't prepared to be led by them anywhere I couldn't see. Sinking deeper into my scatter cushion, my once serene posture crumbled to a pose more associated with the man who sits outside the Underground with the sign 'Wife and three major illnesses to support'. I closed my eyes and prayed to be abducted by Moonies. When the blindfolding had finished, and with no idea who had pinned the tail on the donkey, I paired up with another wild woman for ten minutes of fingertip touching and deep looks. She was laughing more than I was. Maybe she hadn't paid.

As a final act of humiliation, I had to dance out of the labyrinth. Whirling my arms madly to suggest that the day hadn't been a complete loss, I sashayed out of the door. Clicking my heels together three times, I found myself back in Kansas. Three pints of Chardonnay later the shaking subsided. At the risk of bringing on the wrath of the Goddess, where was the sex? Had it all happened in that half an hour when I had mercifully slipped into unconsciousness? My 'Wild Woman' day put me in touch with my wildness only in the sense that it left me totally deranged.

Chapter 12

STAMP DUTY

Realising that my spirit wasn't up to it, I returned to matters of the flesh and, in the process, achieved something that made me feel so proud of myself. In my trophy room, I now had a new honour to put alongside my awards for swimming across the Sea of Galilee and coming first in a Salvation Army test on Leviticus. The certificate read 'This is to certify that Kitty Churchill is a member of The Foot Lover's Appreciation Society'. Just think, me, a member of FLAS! That was one in the eye to the witches at the WI who blackballed me.

Being a member of FLAS entitled me to place an advert in MET-A-TARSAL, the personal column in its magazine. For me this killed two birds with one stone. I'd intended to look at the area of more legitimate lonely hearts and place my own ad. But I have to admit, it was here that my nerve faltered. Men who wrote to complete strangers with a view to foot worship were one thing.

Men who wrote to complete strangers with a view to love were another, and I speak from bitter experience.

It was another Great Idea by Ben. A few years ago, I suffered a particularly long period of manlessness. The damp patch had long since dried up and I started to panic that no-one was ever going to take me down from the shelf for a dust. Ben was getting a little tired of having to dance with me at discos and suggested that I try a lonely hearts column.

'It'll be a laugh,' said Ben.

It wasn't.

Ben helped me compose my ad which went something like, 'Attractive, intelligent, gregarious, left-wing, thirty-year-old woman seeks similar man. Photo appreciated.' (Actually, the one Ben wrote went more like, 'Apolitical, none-too-bright, female lush of indeterminate age, looks passable with dimmer switch, seeks anything in trousers' but I think my precis captured the essence of what he was trying to say.) I received over fifty replies. This had nothing to do with my desirability and everything to do with the fact that the listings magazine in which I'd advertised saw fit to carry my ad for five times longer than the week I'd paid for. Letters from every misfit in London and the Home Counties came flooding in and each week I'd sink into despair as I opened the magazine to find they'd put my advert in again.

One man failed to notice that the same advert had appeared five times. He sent me four letters about his cat. You would think that after four letters I would have been something of an expert on his little feline friend but that wasn't the case. It was the same letter four times over. I didn't worry about how long it took him to write out the same letter again as even the first letter was a photocopy. It was little personal touches like these that made receiving the lonely hearts letters such a joy.

Another man also wrote to me four times but each letter was different. In the first he'd sounded quite nice and had sent a shadowy picture of himself that made him appear fairly decent. I put him on to my 'God, was I drunk last night' pile to deal with after I'd worked through my 'Oh, go on then, seeing as you paid for dinner' pile. Not dealing with him immediately was a wise move. He sent me more letters. The tone in each grew progressively more abusive. He sent another photograph with his final, very aggressive note, demanding that I meet him immediately. This photograph was taken in the sunlight and thinking to myself, 'Darwin was right', I assigned his letters to the 'I've got Mace in my handbag and I've studied ju-jitsu' pile, which was by far the biggest of all.

Some letters were very inventive. I had one which was just a stream of consciousness which, if I hadn't known he was dead, I would have sworn was sent by Jack Kerouac. Another made up a story about me being a princess. Naturally, the writer was my knight in shining armour. I guessed he was a Dungeons and Dragons fan and I Maced him. An ex-monk from Ireland wanted me to take the fear of God out of him, and one man wrote saying that he was involved in an unhappy relationship but couldn't leave until he had somebody else, so would I agree to have an affair with him?

Many sent photographs and for that I was very grateful. The words 'attractive', 'slim' and 'tall' took on completely new meanings. '*The Elephant Man* is my favourite film', 'I'm sure that paving stone was already cracked', and 'You couldn't get those hormone shots when I was growing up', to be precise. One man even told me, as a big plus, he had 'attractive glasses' and sent me a photo of him wearing them to prove his point. They may well have been attractive glasses but since the eyes staring out from behind them belonged to Charles Manson, he went in the Mace pile with the rest of them.

Hope sprang eternal and, finally, I picked out three that had possibilities, reminding myself that, as Ben said, it would be a laugh. And who knew what might happen? I'd seen those Dateline adverts.

My first choice was a solicitor. In the right earning bracket, I thought. He looked quite handsome in his photo and as it was taken in a Photo-Me booth, in all likelihood, he would be much better in the flesh. I arranged to meet him in a wine-bar. Tarted up to the nines (okay, I washed), I breezed into the bar and went into total shock. Wherever that Photo-Me booth was, I wanted to use it. He was to his photo what the newly built Spanish hotel is to the artist's impression in the brochure. It wasn't just that his face looked different – he had no shoulders. He went from ears to hips in a straight line. Telling myself that shoulders aren't every-thing in a man (unless he's a drag queen), I sat down to have a drink with him only to discover he had a rather major speech impediment. It would have taken him hours to say the words 'shoulder pads'. I gave up. I went home and looked at the photograph again and noticed that you could actually see that his whole body fitted inside the edge of the picture.

My next choice was an actor, Pete, who sent me a photo from his portfolio. From his letter, it sounded like we had a lot in common and he looked very pleasant.

Who actually said the camera doesn't lie? Because I'd like to meet that person and slap him. When I met him in a café, I found that Pete had put on four stone since the picture was taken. The excess poundage wasn't so bad but the only thing we had in common was that we'd both come on the bus. I left him my Danish and went home.

I'm five foot four and the third man I met, Mark, barely came up to my armpits. He had a rather bad skin complaint too. If Willie Carson had been working at Chernobyl that day, he might have ended up looking something like Mark. I was determined to have one success from this whole sorry enterprise so, getting drunk, I invited him to my flat.

Back on my settee, barely had my lips grazed against his, when he jumped up to say that he had to go home and walk his dog. It took a lot of pleading and a complete loss of dignity to persuade him to stay. Finally, I managed to coax him into bed. At least now we were the same height. I took off all my clothes but he kept his boxer shorts on. As I went to remove them, he leapt out of bed, looking for something in his bag on the floor. Was it a condom? No, it was his inhaler. The mere thought of me removing his underwear had brought on an asthma attack. I was up all night, not wracked with passion, but worrying about any irregularities in his breathing.

I decided that I couldn't, under any circumstances, do the lonely hearts bit again and so MET-A-TARSAL seemed a godsend. FLAS was run by Dennis of Essex and had been founded in 1990 to, according to their leaflet, 'further the interests of Foot Lovers from all walks of life who just like to adore women's feet, to those who engage in cross-dressing, sole tickling, soft B and D (Bondage and Domination), accelerator pedal pumping, as well as treading or stepping on things and other variations.' (Foot worship is a broad church and FLAS probably has to spread itself a bit thin to accommodate all its variations. The Americans are far more specific with, for instance, a group called Squish who supply magazines and videos for 'crush lovers' featuring 'big barefoot ladies trampling on bugs'.)

Dennis heard the calling and the aim of that calling was to bring foot fetishism out of the closet so that its practitioners could live and enjoy the activity openly with the acceptance of society around them. Because, of course, it is a well-known fact that foot fetishists are amongst the most persecuted groups in the world. Indeed, it is believed that a good proportion of the witches of Salem were Squish centrefolds.

I wanted to know why foot fetishists liked feet. FLAS had members all over the UK and their leaflet claimed that the members came from all economic and social backgrounds. There seemed to be no reason why people would end up this way. I asked Ben (who had come out as a shoe fetishist after his encounter with Paula at the Ring of Confidentes) why he was the way he was. Tossing aside the genetic theory, he felt that it may well have originated in an incident where his mother had hit him over the head with a Dr Scholl.

FLAS said of its personal column 'MET-A-TARSAL': 'We are not a dating service but many of our members are keen to develop foot friendships with others.' And, although FLAS was an overtly sexual society, they were not in the business of providing any kind of pornography. 'We just love FEM-FEET, FEM-FEET and more FEM-FEET! That's our only obsession in life.'

Along with the leaflet, Dennis had sent me a shakily handwritten note telling me how, as a woman, I could get a discount on the £30 membership fee. To get my reduction I had to send off one or more pairs of high heel shoes to 'Choosy Shoesy', FLAS's own stiletto shoe shop. In fact, there was no fee at all if you sent six pairs. I was told that 'most worn shoes can be obtained from Jumble Sales or Charity Shops, if you don't have any'. Having never been First Lady of the Philippines, I went off once again to my favourite deviant's outfitters, Oxfam, and chose a dainty pair of black, size four high heels. The assistant seemed suspicious that I didn't try them on, but one day, if Dennis achieved his goal, she'd understand.

I posted off the shoes and £15 to Choosy Shoesy and a couple of days later, I received my certificate (I still get a rush of pride even now), the club magazine, *Footsy*, and another spidery note from Dennis. He was slightly confused as to why I'd joined as FLAS did not have a preponderance of single female members. Which just goes to show how much shame people still feel about this perfectly normal way of life. Dennis said, if I wanted to, that I could write a letter on the other side of the foot/shoe point of view which would be printed in the magazine. He wanted to know if I had attractive feet. If so, could I let him have a fotoe and then I could be in with a chance of being the *Footsy* centrefold and claim my '*Footsy* Feature Fee'. Dennis signed off with 'your Footmate'. I resolved to send off a pedi-picture just as soon as the cornplasters came off.

A copy of *Footsy* magazine wouldn't shame even the

most sophisticated of coffee tables, although at £6 for non-members per bi-monthly issue, it wasn't cheap. The front cover hinted at the delights inside showing pictures of three pairs of women's feet and the headlines:

Ladies barefeet

Nylon stockings and high-heeled shoes

Femdom feet.

I hurriedly turned to the Big Toe editorial to find out how Dennis was coping with the stresses of his important mission. Apparently, one of the Footsy staff writers had left, no doubt burnt out by all that campaigning. But the good news was that she had been replaced by Auntie Claire. Said Dennis, 'She has such big feet – lovely size eights – and do they smell, real cheesy . . . and from what I can tell she is going to make sure I toe-the-line or else? (So nice to have a dominant woman with big feet to step on things when they get behind)'. If Dennis upset Auntie Claire, he would have to 'get down and suck and lick her smelly cheesy feet'. I hoped that irregular question mark occasioned at least a mouthful of toe.

The next page featured a picture of Auntie Claire in all her size eight glory. Her opening gambit was, 'My dear Cheesy Stilton *toe suckers*'. Auntie was offering her old nylons, socks and slippers for sale and was also intending to feetpose in the privacy of her own 'Toeture Chamber'. One person had even asked for her toenail clippings which, in a fit of magnanimity, she had duly sent. I couldn't even begin to think what the lucky recipient intended to do with them. Auntie finished off her introductory piece talking about her foot slaves and rolling her feet around in cauliflower cheese (no recipe provided).

I would have thought the likes of Curtess and Clarks

would be fighting over the advertising space in *Footsy*. Again, I think this is something that will come in time when foot love emerges from the closet (or in this case, pump bag). There were, however, extensive ads placed by The American Gina Lang Collection which showed women licking each other's toes. My chequebook quivered in anticipation as I scanned through the Gina Lang photolist. 'Amber is captured by two female ticklers. She is dressed in pantyhose and a bathing suit. She is tickled and then forced to her knees to lick the foot of one lady. Amber has Bruce massage her feet with his fingers and mouth. Her bare feet and pretty painted toes get his complete attention. Great footworship close ups.' When Amber had to put her feet up, Nicole, Kelly and Meg were ready to step into her shoes.

After '*TOES-R-US*' (more pictures of women's feet being tickled and licked, this time from the American magazine *Beautiful Bare Feet*), Dennis did an in-depth report on the feet-tickling scene in America. It made me sad to think that there was a place in this world where the right to bare feet was protected by the Constitution. Humming a bar from 'We Shall Overcome', I finished the piece and noted Dennis's request for information from anyone who knew how to build laughing stocks as Texas Homecare were right out.

There were more photos in Pat's Peds. In a couple of pictures Patricia had coyly placed her stiletto over her naked crotch. At the bottom of the page it read, 'To fantasize about licking a Dominant woman's feet is, for most, only a fantasy. It's something to dream about. For the lucky footslave who sent in these fotoes of his mistress, every so often fantasy becomes reality when he is ordered to worship Madam's damp sweaty feet. The

aroma is fantastic, especially when she has been shopping all day wearing these stockings and high heels. Her
slave is forced to lick the salty taste of fresh sweat from
behind her toes, knowing if he does not satisfy her he
will be spanked hard and not allowed to return to his
fantasy for some time to come. Pat has made that quite
clear to her footslaves.'

I noted from the magazine that the foot worshipper
did not discriminate. No arch was too fallen, no nail
polish too chipped that it would be denied a place in the
Footsy pantheon. The foot lover is possessed of that rare
quality – unconditional foot love. These people were at
the vanguard of a new era of understanding. The sweep
and compassion of the footworshipping movement left
one in awe. Dennis made Martin Luther King look like
a man complaining at a bus-stop.

I must confess I didn't read the fiction section or any
of the foot lover's stories and only perused through the
letters page which were all written by men, as by now I
was feeling a bit footigued (obviously I'm getting the
hang-nail of the lingo). Especially as there were still fifteen pages to go and many more photos of feet. I was
slightly disappointed by the quality of the cartoon strip,
Solemates. The artist was Gal and Gal had obviously
drawn it holding the pencil between his (?) toes.
Accompanying a drawing of a woman shoving a trainer
in a kneeling man's face, was the caption, 'Look, stupid,
smell right inside, taste and smell, do you still like my
smelly feet? I think you do, your (sic) so hard and
twitching down there . . .' and so on.

I sadly came to the end of the magazine. The last item
was called Toetal Defeet, and for a change showed pictures of women sucking other women's toes. I'll confess,

it left me hot. My corns throbbed as I rushed off and posted my own small ad: 'Very stern meter maid seeks fallen-arch supporters to park her rank size sixes on'. My Footsy ad appeared in the next issue, slightly amended by Auntie Claire so that 'Very stern' became 'Lovely Rita'. I went out and bought a pumice stone and waited for the replies to come flooding in.

I didn't get a single letter. Do you think that the gentlemen of The Foot Lover's Appreciation Society thought I was a prostoetute?

Chapter 13

LOVE THAT'S ONLY SLIGHTLY SOILED

I wondered if women got a better class of man if they paid for it. Alec was a male escort whose number I'd found in the back of the women's soft porn magazine *For Women*. Over the phone he told me that he charged £20 for a massage and another £50 if I required 'extras'.

'How long do the extras last?' I asked.

'Every lady is unique,' Alec answered. 'Do you want the "O"?'

'I'll have to think about it.'

To be completely honest, I didn't know which 'O' he meant, orgasm or oral, although I didn't really care as I wasn't about to pay anything for a man who called women, 'ladies'. You just knew he'd put the word 'foxy' in front of it given half a chance.

The second escort I tried didn't give his name in the advert.

'I want to talk to you about hiring your services,' I said, nervously.

He sounded around forty-five years old and was charm itself. 'Are you winding me up? I'm bloody sick of these crank calls.'

I assured him that I was genuinely in need of his attentions and asked him his name.

'Mark Anthony,' he said. 'What's yours?'

'Cleopatra,' I replied to lighten the mood.

'You are winding me up. I've had enough of this.'

I calmed him down for five minutes and then told him that I wanted to meet him in a pub first so that I could vet him.

He took some persuading, then finally agreed. 'But I'm not dressing up for you. Some women want you to wear a dinner-suit and all that gear. But I won't do it.'

He asked me how he'd recognise me.

'I'll be wearing a leather jacket.'

'Ooer, that's kinky,' said Mark Anthony, man of the world, then added, 'I charge £10 an hour, minimum six hours.'

He then agreed that for this initial meeting, his time could be bought for a pint.

The thought of spending six hours with Mark Anthony shunting away on top of me was enough to send me reaching for the asp. Fortunately, our meeting was never to be. He rang me at midnight that same evening, having insisted that I give him my phone number to prove that it wasn't a wind-up. He was very drunk and belligerent.

'Why d'ya phone me?' he slurred.

'I just wanted to know what it would be like to hire a man.' I told him I didn't appreciate being rung so late in the evening.

'I couldn't talk to you properly before,' he explained, 'because I was in the car with my uncle. I'm not used to this mobile phone either. I could be in the kharzi taking a leak when someone rings.'

Bowled over by his magnetism, I let him rant on about how, ever since he put the advert in, he had received no end of crank calls from women wanting freebie obscene phonecalls. I made the right sympathetic noises but pointed out that that was the risk of advertising.

He wasn't mollified. 'And another thing. How come you get to vet me first but I'm expected to say I'll go with you sight unseen?'

I was exasperated. 'This is your job. We're talking about an economic transaction here. It is normal for the customer to see the merchandise before buying.'

'But you might walk away when you see me.'

I know that honesty is a voguish approach to advertising but Mark Anthony wasn't selling himself too well. I tried to get him off the phone saying that there was no point in us meeting as it all appeared to be too much hassle. Mark Anthony, however, wasn't letting what was probably the closest thing he'd ever had to a genuine offer off the hook that easily. He began to insist that I meet him, but his demands were cut short when the battery on his mobile phone failed.

Later in the night he left another message on my answer phone which I ignored. He then had the nerve to call me again the next morning to see if our meeting was still on. I put the phone down on him and called *For Women* to make a complaint.

Mark Anthony had confirmed some of my hunches about escorts for women. I suspected that the types advertising to be paid were probably the sort that couldn't give it away for free. Although there had been an explosion of media interest in male escorts over the previous months, I was beginning to think that the only people who actually rang them were other journalists. Indeed, a producer from the BBC got my number from *For Women* to see if I wanted to be interviewed about using escorts as they'd been unable to track down any other women who admitted they did.

Chastened by the experience, I thought about leaving the subject of hiring a man alone. But looking at the escorts page again with a very jaundiced eye, I noticed one advert for a male stripper. It read: 'A professional, good-looking male stripper will strip for you and much, much more!! Just call Sebastian.'

Sebastian also pointed out that he was the magazine's man of the month and could be seen on page eighty-six in all of his naked splendour. I turned to the spread indicated which was entitled 'Roman Holiday'. A well-lubricated Sebastian was posing nude in front of a Doric column in the time honoured classical tradition. He had the body of David but, unfortunately, the penis of David's six-year-old brother, Japeth. But hiring a stripper was almost like hiring an escort and inviting some friends around to see him meant there'd be safety in numbers. Besides, I consoled myself, I could always offer to pay him by the inch.

So I phoned Sebastian to book him for my hen night.

'What does "much, much more" mean?' I asked.

'What do you want it to mean?' he replied in a sexy foreign accent.

I wanted it to mean much, much more than he was showing off in the photographs but I said nothing.

Sebastian charged £60 for a twenty-minute performance in front of an all-girl audience which came in at
about £35 an inch. He said that for another £10 he was
prepared to do his act for a mixed crowd. Earlier, I'd
shown Roman Holiday to Ben and his only comment
was a sniffy, 'Obviously a winter holiday', so I thought
the extra tenner would be wasted.

Although ordering a stripper was easier than phoning
for a pizza, finding an appreciative audience proved
problematic. None of my women friends wanted to come
and see a man take off his clothes in my living-room. I
don't think any of them were convinced that I'd really
hire somebody. I think they just thought I'd put 'Wheels
Cha-Cha' on my CD and Ben would appear in a thong.
And they'd all seen that at countless parties before. I had
to send round the Roman Holiday pictures before any of
them would agree to come and even then they phoned
up with comments like, 'Make sure you've got the heating on' and 'Remind me to bring my reading glasses'.

On the night, I packed Dominic off to the pub, asking
him to hit the central heating switch on his way out. I'd
booked Sebastian for nine o'clock and he said he would
arrive twenty minutes before that in order to get ready,
although he wouldn't elaborate on what that entailed.
Now, I've read about 'fluffers' who work in the porn
film industry so I thought it might be something like
that. Fluffers are off-screen technicians whose job it is to
make sure that the male stars remain at full stretch.
Therefore, to keep the continuity, the fluffer must 'fluff'
(orally or manually) the star's acting credentials in
between takes. So I had some Listermint and a pair of
Marigolds at the ready just in case.

At nine o'clock, there were seven women in my

living-room getting twitchy and no sign of Sebastian. Initially, they had been nervous, but now they were ready for anything Sebastian could throw at them, which from Roman Holiday didn't look likely to be anything that would leave a permanent mark. He finally arrived at gone half past, having got lost on the way. He was about six feet tall with a chiselled, classical face, lovely green eyes and very short dark hair. He was looking good, but nothing like he did in the photographs. He was carrying a large holdall containing his stage clothes and I directed him up to my bedroom to change.

Back in the living-room, the girls were getting impatient.

'It's worth waiting for,' I said, even though they'd already seen it and knew that it wasn't.

Just then Sebastian called me from the hall. 'Kitty, I need your help.'

I stood up and cracked my knuckles. I was ready to fluff.

Out in the hallway, Sebastian was dressed from head to foot in leather. His leather waistcoat revealed his muscular arms and chest. His leather chaps showed off his pert bum and a studded cod piece shielded his disappointment. He held out a tape and told me to play it.

'And . . .' I said expectantly.

'Make sure you turn the volume right up.'

I went back into the living-room and turned on the tape machine. If the girls laughed at it, it would be nobody's fault but his own.

As the intro to Madonna's 'Erotica' boomed out, the girls weren't laughing at anybody. Suddenly overcome by coyness, they were all trying to hide behind each other on the sofa. Bumping and grinding, Sebastian entered the room. The reception was lukewarm. Sensing that the crowd weren't yet on his side, Sebastian shook his booty harder and, at the climax of the song, jumped into the air and landed in the splits. The room was silent aside from Sheila telling Caron how sore her nipples were from breast feeding.

The music started again. Sebastian took off his waist-coat and grabbed Caron, pushing his groin into her face. He then made Sheila rub baby oil over his chest. She wasn't fazed as she'd been up to her armpits in baby oil all day anyway. Everybody had to have a go at the oil routine and I feared for the plush of my soft furnishings. Reaching Fran, one of the only women there who had actually been keen to come, he picked her up, wrapped her legs around his waist and began dipping her. Unfortunately, he dipped too low and she hit her head on the floorboards. Pausing briefly to apologise, Sebastian leapt on top of her and pumped up and down between her legs.

The look on Betty's face warned off Sebastian from trying any of that funny business with her and he merely tangoed around the room with her for a minute. He then picked up Rose and held her above his head. Rose is a very demure, quiet woman and had only come as a special favour to me. She also stands six feet tall in her stockings, so it was no mean feat on Sebastian's part when he lifted her up, wrapped her legs around his face and went into a spin. As she screamed it occurred to me that the muslin drapes I have up at the front room window hide nothing from the street.

As the rest of the audience seemed to be either con-cussed or lactating, Sebastian concentrated his attentions on me. He sat me on a chair in the middle of the room, blindfolded me and handcuffed my hands.

Sitting astride me, he pulled my hands down to touch something between his legs which was big, hard, oily and strapped on. He then shoved this dildo into my mouth. I gagged so he withdrew and made me masturbate the strap-on which poured out more baby oil appreciatively.

Untied, I skidded back to my seat. He danced out of his chaps and tried to make Fran kneel in front of him. She was still seeing stars and having none of it. He cajoled but she refused point blank to take off his codpiece. Sebastian seemed perplexed, wondering why he had been hired when nobody actually wanted to see him take off his clothes. He was forced to take off the codpiece himself, revealing a very small G-string. Here it comes, I thought, the big let down.

'This is for you,' he said to Fran, thrusting his G-string dangerously close to her face. But, unless he had a box of Nurofen in there as well, Fran didn't want it.

Seeing that I was the only one in the slightest bit interested, he came over to me and whipped off his G-string treating me to a close-up of his semi-hard penis. It looked nothing like the one in the picture. Finishing his act, he kissed each of us in turn and was away to put his clothes on again.

Although everyone agreed he'd been very professional, nobody had found it the least bit erotic. I should have stuck with Ben after all. He isn't erotic either but he does know how to get baby oil out of linen. When Sebastian came down again, dressed, I showed him the Roman Holiday pictures.

'It didn't look like it does here,' I said, by way of showing my appreciation.

I felt a bit stupid when he said, 'That's because it isn't

mine' and explained that he'd been man of a different month.

I told Sebastian about my lack of success with escorts and as luck would have it, he said that he did escort work too. Having already fingered the merchandise, I booked him for another night. Just to talk, mind.

When Dominic found out that Sebastian was not 'Roman Holiday' but 'Free! Naked Man', he wasn't so easy to get out of the house. Fortunately, Ben had a domestic crisis when his ex came by to try and retrieve some of his consumer durables from Ben's flat. Dominic had to rush over to stop him taking it out on the little crockery he had left. Settling down with a bottle of wine, I read through Sebastian's particulars. I was delighted to find that, although he was only twenty-four, he had a taste for older women, naming Faye Dunaway as his favourite. I phoned Ben to see if he had calmed down and to check that Dominic was really out of the way.

'Do you think that I'm as attractive as Faye Dunaway is nowadays?' I asked.

'Try Fay Wray,' he replied and slammed down the phone.

I knew Dominic would be fully occupied all evening.

Sebastian had agreed to talk to me for £60, a considerable drop from the £200 he'd charged a women's magazine for an interview the week before. I was delighted by the concession but, yet again, it confirmed my belief that the only people paying for escorts are journalists.

I'd finished the bottle of wine by the time Sebastian arrived. He didn't drink but rolled a joint instead. Sebastian claimed in his man of the month slot that he was a jeans and T-shirt man and only dressed up for special occasions. As he was wearing a dog-tooth check jacket, a black polo neck and black trousers, I thought: Faye Dunaway, and hummed a few bars of 'Windmills of my Mind'.

Sebastian told me that he had been stripping for two years and had recently decided to bump up his income by becoming an escort. I wanted to know why women would pay to have sex with a man when it's quite easy to get it for free. Sebastian admitted that this was a problem but he did now have a client whom he was sleeping with several nights a week. Unfortunately, Sebastian was one of those creatures of myth – a tart with a heart – and his sliding scale of payment meant that, after an initial sixty pounds a session, he was now down to ten pounds a night with his client.

She had been hurt by a former lover and, after a string of one-night stands, had become very depressed, losing her sense of self-worth. Somehow, she had decided that hiring a male escort for the night would restore her confidence and dignity. The first escort sent to her was a scruffy looking fifty-year-old who arrived on her doorstep with a carrier bag full of sex aids. (I mentioned the name Mark Anthony but it didn't ring any bells.) She wouldn't even let him in the door and, from the threshold, he begged her to let him have sex with her. She refused but, amazingly, she decided to give another escort a go. She got Sebastian and, understandably, they had sex immediately.

'She only lives ten minutes from me. So it's handy and she takes me out to nice places,' said Sebastian. 'She likes the arrangement because, as long as she pays, I'll always be there for her. When I'm paid, I like to treat a woman right.'

But it seemed that this client was the exception. The main reason why women hired Sebastian was to get back at ex-lovers. An advertising executive had taken him to a party to prove to her ex-fiancé that she was fine and could have a young stud dangling off her arm if she chose. Another jilted woman hired him to seduce her ex-boyfriend's new girlfriend. The new girlfriend was a hairdresser and the jilted woman planned to take photographs of Sebastian with the crimper and show them to her ex. Sebastian booked in for a haircut, tipped generously and sent a bunch of flowers a few days later, asking for a date. Unfortunately, the hairdresser was totally in love and spurned Sebastian's advances. Feeling he had failed his client, he offered to sleep with her for free. She contemplated the idea but decided it wasn't the answer.

Sebastian said that he charged £30 for a one-to-one strip and the same price for a massage.

'What do you get with your massage?' I asked, hunching my shoulders.

'If the woman was relaxed, I would masturbate her. Some come in ten minutes.'

He came and sat next to me on the settee and began massaging my back. It felt extremely good but I decided I'd better stop it as Dominic had taken my cash card.

Sebastian moved and sat opposite me, smiling.

'What are you thinking?' I asked.

'About how last night I couldn't sleep for thinking about you.'

If I didn't know this was costing me £60, I would have bought it. Instead, I asked him how he managed to perform if the woman was really unattractive.

'I wouldn't sleep with her.'

'That would destroy her if she couldn't even get sex when she was paying for it,' I said.

'Okay. I would charge her more.'

'What if you couldn't get an erection?'

'There are tricks of the trade,' he said, fishing out an elastic band from his pocket. 'I get myself hard and then wrap this around my cock and balls and it keeps me going.'

I asked him what he did in bed.

'Anything, apart from anal sex. But every woman is different. I give it to them the way they like it. I believe I am selling energy. Sex is energy. It's just another commodity.'

I wanted to tell him that I intended to buy shares immediately, but I couldn't as, completely stoned, I had to rush off to the bathroom to throw up.

Owing to the drink and dope, I'm afraid I lost all journalistic credibility and professionalism. I came back from the bathroom and knocked over a glass of wine (which Sebastian graciously mopped up) and told him more about my sex life than he ever told me about his. He did reveal that he'd become an escort partly because he'd had to do national service in his native country.

'In the army you have to do what everybody else tells you to. I wanted to be my own person and do what I wanted, when I wanted.'

And with that he came and sat next to me again and resumed the massage. Then he started to kiss me. Pulling myself away, which took a lot of will-power, I told him that I was much too egotistical ever to pay for sex.

'I'm not charging you,' he said, moving towards me again.

At that precise moment, Dominic walked through the front door.

Nearly.

Chapter 14

PLASTERED

'I'm sorry, I've lost it,' said Dominic.

After Sebastian, Dominic had felt a little bit left out and I tried to make it up to him by asking him to participate in my next assignment. But men! Honestly! Ask them to do one simple thing like maintain an erection while you dunk it into a cut-off Fairy Liquid bottle filled with plaster of Paris and they go to pieces on you. He wouldn't have had to do it if Big John had arrived . . .

I had sent away for an inflatable man which was advertised in the back of a sex magazine. For only £19.95, Big John came complete with two orifices and a vibrating penis. After waiting the regulation twenty-eight days, I admitted to myself that Big John had stood me up. Let me tell you, just because a man needs the attentions of a bicycle pump to inflame his ardour, it doesn't mean you can't still feel the rejection when he doesn't show. He could have at least phoned. I'd spent that month planning what

I was going to use the two orifices for. Ashtrays seemed as good as anything.

Most sex toys seem to be made in China and it's no wonder they've clung to Communism when the average factory worker must believe that Capitalism leads to a need for Big John dolls. John had a sister whose name was Talking Laura. The advert read (and it may have lost something in the translation), 'She has beautiful blonde hair and a very curvy body. She is ready for all kinds of unusual positions that you can think of. She has a mouth, vagina and anus. She has a powerful mouth pump that will give ultra sensation to your vital part. She can also make lusty noise to increase that realistic feeling.' Talking Laura sounded like a hoover with a wig on.

But why bother with all those non-essentials like arms, legs, heads and torsos when you can just buy the business end? The 'Natural Pussy', which came in both vibrating and still versions, was a 'luxurious imitation with fine pubic hair, vaginal lips and clitoris'. I wasn't too impressed by the fine pubic hair as, from what I could see in the picture, the Natural Pussy seemed to be suffering from a touch of alopecia. And, as many men don't bother with clitorises normally, I wondered what they would do with a plastic one.

Of the numerous penis imitations for women, none came with fine pubic hair. Many didn't even look like the real thing. The 'Real Feel Bear' had a totem pole shaped shaft that 'twists and squirms tantalisingly'. There was a little bear jutting out from its side, which, believe it or not, was a clitoral stimulator. The bear was capable, apparently, of sending one into a sexual frenzy. One for those Christopher Robin moments, I felt.

If I was going for dismembered parts, I wanted to get

as near to the real things as possible; which was how Dominic came to be attached to a Fairy Liquid bottle. The product was called, rather poetically, 'The Mould-A-Willy Kit'. I spent an inordinately long time waiting for this to arrive too. When it did, it was clear that the packaging had been tampered with. About this time, I noticed that the postman had begun whistling 'It's Just on the Street Where You Live' when he delivered the mail. Was Big John not the man I thought he was?

The Mould-A-Willy Kit came from a company that also sold vibrators in the shape of various foodstuffs. Why somebody would want to turn themselves on with a twenty-three-inch baguette was beyond me. But then, maybe some women think of Percy Ingles as an erogenous zone.

The advert said, 'Replicate the willy of your choice as a rubber vibrator. It's easy . . . it's fun!' I think I could report them to the Advertising Standards Authority over that one. In the first place, Dominic and I had a slight disagreement over which willy I should replicate. I, Cynthia Plastercaster, was all in favour of a baguette-sized ex-boyfriend as the kit cost the same as Big John and I wanted to get my money's worth. Ben offered his services but I thought there are some things friends shouldn't do for each other and, anyway, I think he was confusing metric with imperial. Dominic won out in the end. I couldn't help thinking that although I was meant to be trying out what was going on in other people's bedrooms, there was no-one else in the country stupid enough to be moulding a willy.

The kit contained one pot of latex, one moulding vessel, one vibrator, one sheet of release film, one paintbrush and one bag of moulding plaster. The quality was not high. The release film was a tatty old bit of cling-film probably straight off a sandwich which was holding together a split, plastic beaker which, I assumed, was the moulding vessel. This vessel, said the instructions, 'will suit the average man, but members of the big boys club will have to use a washing-up liquid bottle with the top cut off!' Dominic went straight off to cut up a bottle. I didn't have the heart to point out that it was a Fairy Excel Plus bottle.

The first instruction was to 'make a hole through the release film with your finger and then push your erect member through it. Wrap the release film around your testicles . . . (Be sure not to mould your pubic hair, it's painful when taking it off.) Don't worry about getting plaster on your willy – it releases when you lose the erec-tion and washes off.' There were diagrams too, for those who felt that these instructions weren't explicit enough. Once shrink-wrapped, you had to mix the plaster and fill up the moulding vessel. 'You then have approximately two minutes or until the plaster turns jellylike to regain the largest stiffy of your life! Holding the moulding pot upright, bend over and plunge your stiffy into the pot . . . Concentrate on keeping your stiffy.'

(I would like to say at this point, that my advice to any women reading this and excited by the thought of pur-chasing their own Mould-A-Willy Kit, is that they would be better off standing on their heads and filling them-selves up with plaster as at least that way they would be assured of producing something that fits.)

'Think Nanette Newman,' I said, as Dominic plunged into the Fairy Liquid bottle. Maybe Dominic was worried what Bryan Forbes would think; it didn't work. It was like trying to mix concrete with a daffodil. Ignoring the plaster on the bathroom floor, he made a second attempt. This was no better. Dominic lost his erection as soon as it went into the bottle. His pride was dented more than the plaster. I was quite keen still to cast the result in latex but Dominic said that there was no way he was going to allow me to parade a two inch dildo shaped like a fish hook in front of my friends and say it was him. We then had an argument about who was going to clean up the bathroom floor. I binned the Mould-A-Willy Kit. It wasn't easy and it wasn't fun.

Maybe my choice of the Mould-A-Willy Kit was just too esoteric. A week or so after that tragic experience, I was in Ann Summers in Charing Cross Road leafing through a copy of *Shaven Ravers*, the magazine for depilation enthusiasts, when two things hit me. One was, that if I was looking for the average sex aid for the average person in England, then Ann Summers was the ideal place to look. The other thing was that Flo, forty-eight, housewife and shaven raver, should let it all grow back as it looked like the 'Natural Pussy'.

When Thinking of England, Ann Summers is right up there with Madame Tussauds, crap sitcoms and rain: quintessentially English. I couldn't really creep around after shoppers to look in their baskets to see what they were buying so I got myself invited to an Ann Summers party. I received the invite through a friend of a friend so I didn't really know any of the women that were going. It worked better that way. Most of my friends are sexually well beyond the level where Ann Summers could be of any assistance and, if I'd held a party, the hostess would be lucky to earn enough commission for her bus fare. Now if Ann Summers introduced a Black & Decker range, it would be a different matter.

Ann Summers parties are strictly women-only affairs. This one was held by Sue for eight of her friends, all in their early twenties, in her council flat on the tenth floor of a tower block. By the time I arrived they were raring to go. The hostess, Gloria, a big woman in her mid-thirties, felt the proceedings had to be warmed up even further by beginning with a couple of party games. The prizes were either a Mr Willy notepad or a bottle of Booby Drops which came in three flavours to enhance the taste of one's nipples and drive men crazy. These were Wild Cherry, Strawberry & Pineapple and Lager. I took a raincheck on the games. Dominic likes a drink but I think even he'd blanch if I presented him with a breast smacking of Heineken.

The others showed no such reticence. The first game involved writing down imaginary sexual problems and providing their solutions. The questions and answers were shuffled and so, in reply to a query on frigidity, the answer would read, 'Dear Long Lips, I'm afraid the only solution is scissors or clamps'. In the middle of this game, one of the women's baby daughter started crying and the mother briefly entertained the idea of giving her a vibrator to pacify her. The reply to 'Horny and Hairy' got lost as the subject turned to baby wipes and milk expressors.

Gloria expertly brought things back to the matter in hand and introduced game two, 'the quickest blow job and the fastest orgasm', which, she delightedly told everybody, was her own invention. The game required a balloon, a pump and four willing thighs. 'Harder, harder,' screamed the pumpees as the pumpers shunted away behind them. The climax of the game entailed sitting on the balloon and shouting 'orgasm'. A brief refractory period was then allowed whilst the winners pocketed their Mr Willy notepads.

Flushed and panting, the women were ready for the hard sell. Gloria introduced the Ann Summers lingerie collection. We oohed at the 'Malandra' ('Feminine corselet with lace V panel') and we aahed at the 'Faye' ('Stretch lace G-string body-hugger'). Then we came to the 'Kimberley' ('Luxurious teddy with stretch-lace panel and French-knicker-style brief with crotch fastening') and while Gloria confessed that the 'Kimberley' wasn't supportive to the fuller figure, the women discussed the pros and cons of fiddling with a press stud gusset when going for a wee. The consensus of opinion was that it was okay merely to hold the gusset to one side whilst peeing, though this made it difficult to pull off a piece of toilet paper with only one hand.

Although the 'Kimberley' couldn't take a full load, Ann Summers does produce a range of 'Sensual Styles for the Fuller Figure' called the 'Twice As Sexy' range. And good on them too, I thought, marvelling at the amount of fabric that went into a size 24 'Rhonda'. Gloria ploughed through seemingly endless combinations of underwired and overstretched lingerie, each garment with a more exotic name tag than the last. The 'Foxy', the 'Blaze', the 'Pandora', the 'Prunella' – on and on they came. I was knickered. None of these undergarments were the slightest bit raunchier than the drawers on sale in M&S.

The clothing from the 'Erotica' catalogue was nearer the mark, featuring as it did toned-down fetishwear such as his and hers leather harnesses. We are led to believe that an interest in fetishwear is something of a fringe taste and yet Ann Summers aims its goods right at the middle of the market. The women at the party seemed more interested in this catalogue than all that had gone before and I would guess that none of them would ever dream of going to Torture Garden.

There's a good reason why Ann Summers parties are women only – men wouldn't stand a chance. The goods on sale are biased towards flattering and glamorising women while laughing at the sexuality of men. When Gloria said we had forgotten the chaps, there was a chorus of, 'Why do you think we're here buying vibrators'. A good example of this attitude was the 'Ankle Penis'.

'This is for men who like to show off,' said Gloria. 'They simply attach it to their ankles and then nonchalantly pull up their trouser leg.'

The women couldn't care less. They'd come for vibrators and vibrators they were going to have. Three of the vibrators in particular stuck in my mind and made me think that maybe the Mould-A-Willy wasn't quite so odd after all. The 'Foreskin' was a 'sensational 8½ inch vibrator with realistic skin movement'. I wasn't keen and picked up a circumcised model. This one talked.

'Come on bubby, give it to me harder. Oh, God, that feels good. Give it to me harder. Oh, yeah,' said the vibrator.

I put it down. The other women agreed with me that the point of having a vibrator was that it didn't answer back.

Finally, Gloria pulled the 'Emperor' out of her bag and there was a collective intake of breath. Eight inches long, easily as wide and complete with an impressive set of balls, the Emperor also had the bonus of a sucker attached to the bottom.

'This allows you,' said Gloria, 'to stick it on to your coffee-table, which leaves your hands free for something else.'

Free for phoning an ambulance, I thought, looking at the monster, but Sue was keen to attach it to her washing machine to give it a go on spin cycle.

I didn't find out what the other women bought, which was the point of the exercise. When it came to ordering, the women suddenly became very quiet. I'm quite sure some of them went away having spent £35 on an Emperor, but if they did they weren't saying. And what about me? Did I succumb to the Rhonda or the Foreskin? I'm not saying, either. But I will admit to leaving Sue's flat with a prominent bulge beneath the cuff of my jeans . . .

Chapter 15

Better Than Peters And Lee?

Miss Sugar Cane had done an admirable job of shimmying out of her dress to reveal that her knickers were still in her underwear drawer. But as she spun around to give the punters a chance to look at her spotlit behind, she smacked her face into the six-foot cardboard cake iced with the words, 'Thirty-Five Years Of Raymond's Revue'. With her blonde Marilyn wig only slightly askance, she finished her routine to the rapturous applause of the mainly Japanese audience. I was having my last night out with Ben before my wedding. Of course, I managed to combine it with my sexual investigation so we were doing Soho, and the climax of the evening was a visit to 'The Festival of Erotica'.

'If we're going up West,' said Ben before we went out, 'you've got to wear the coney.'

It was one of those rare occasions when I knew exactly

what he meant. Despite gentrification and the development of the area as a gay village over the last few years, Soho still has that allure of faded glamour and naughty-but-niceness that needs a cheap fur coat and a spangly dress to do a visit there justice. But I knew that, on our evening out, we would be visiting a porn cinema and it would be pretty hard to explain to my mother why there was a bank manager's emission laced across the detachable collar of her only fur coat.

We started our evening by checking out a few of the sex shops. Once, as research for an article, I had accompanied one of Westminster Council's Licensing Officers on a tour around Soho. He told me that, for a bookshop to be deemed a sex shop and therefore need a licence, a significant degree of the material on sale must be of a sexual nature. This explains why, when you walk into most of the sex shops in Soho, you have to wade through stacks of remaindered copies of Baden-Powell's biography or *The Guide to State Schools 1971* before you see even a hint of nipple.

Hardcore porn was available in most of the shops that we went into. That is to say the covers of the magazines were hardcore, but as they were mostly sealed in shrinkwrap it was difficult to know if the contents were of the strength promised by the cover. It isn't unknown for unscrupulous vendors to remove the covers of hardcore magazines and staple them to magazines which contain nothing more obscene than the contents of an average issue of the *National Geographic*.

There must be a DIY book entitled *Soho Interiors*, as the layouts of the shops worked to a formula. First and foremost, at the door, there is the ubiquitous multi-coloured fly curtain, passing through which transports the customer from the drear of the normal world into a land of wonder in much the same way as going into the wardrobe does in the Narnia books. Only this is no land of permanent winter and power-mad witches, but one of permanent tumescence and 'sex-crazed bitches'.

For, once you've decided that your life will be in no way improved by a dog-eared copy of *Decimalisation Made Easy*, you can move on to the punchboard-backed MDF shelves groaning under the weight of magazines which show stiffened members, of a colour never seen in nature, sunk to the scrotum in gaping and similarly-hued vaginas. Invariably, the women in these photographs will, with two badly nail-polished fingers in a V-shape, be holding back their labia to allow the camera a better shot of the penis, which invariably belongs to a man with Georgie Best sideburns, going about its business. Likewise, one of the fingers on the other hand of the recipient of all this love action will be resting on the tip of her tongue which protrudes through her slightly parted red-lipsticked lips in an expression which signifies to pornophiles, the world over, that the woman is experiencing a moment of almost transcendental ecstasy.

Aside from the magazines and a shelf of similarly illus-trated videos, there is normally a display case filled with what may be dildoes and vibrators but what could just as easily be the contents of a salad drawer, as the level of dust covering the objects makes positive identification difficult to ascertain. Brave is the woman, indeed, who would sit on one of these objects without first subjecting it to the attentions of a sandblaster.

Having made your selection from this array of top-notch merchandise, you will queue behind a man wearing a rain mac, despite the hosepipe-ban going on outside, who has a copy of *Popping Mamas* (a magazine for enthusiasts of naked, third trimester mothers-to-be) under his arm and who is sweating to such an extent that you are prepared to accept the male menopause as a scientific fact. Once he has paid for his goods, placed them in his plastic briefcase and left, you will come face to face with the shop assistant whose hopes of a brilliant career were dashed on the day he flunked his entrance exam for the Burger Academy. This is a man who has no use for pornography himself, as holding a copy of *Jugs* in one hand and running his finger under the words with the other, sadly leaves him a fist short.

The Westminster Licensing Officer told me that when they confiscate stuff, they have a checklist they tick to detail the contents of the material. The list goes something like: buggery, cunnilingus, ejaculation, fellatio, intercourse, masturbation, nudity, sex aids and miscellaneous. If all the sex shops were like the Janus bookshop which we visited, this list would become redundant, as the shop thoughtfully divides its magazines into specialist areas. As sex shops go, it was one of the more pleasant to be in. Although stopping short of using the ISBN classification system, there were sections devoted to transvestism, dominant women, corporal punishment, rubber and leather and, the reason for our visit, wet and messy fun.

Ben wanted to buy a magazine called *Splosh* which covers the 'tapioca in my knickers' scene. He briefly deliberated over a copy of *Rocky Mountain High* which showed two male mountaineers enjoying more than a yodel, before shelling out £7 for *Splosh* in order to look at the pictorials on:

Food flies at our Lady Mayor's messy fête

Denise and Dawn – dirty mud fight

Keystone kapers: our WPC cops the pies!

As a break from our investigation, we went to a pub so that Ben could check out his purchase. Like so many of the other fetishes I'd come across, the erotic appeal of looking at a picture of a woman having a tin of Bird's Custard poured over her brassière was totally beyond me. The magazine has a devoted following and is something of a cult. Said Steven from Cardiff on the letters page, regarding a previous issue, 'Samantha-Jane looks as cheeky as ever . . . Yet again she treats us to the delightful sight of her panties full of food. Karen really looks like she's enjoying every minute and her cleavage holds enough syrup to drown in. And there's Robyn . . . The photograph [of her] sitting on a chair with her panties full of rice pudding is my new favourite . . .'

I looked briefly at the picture spread showing the Lady Mayoress having Calthwaite's low fat yoghurt poured over her head by Jackie the saucy stallholder at a village fête (economically held in somebody's back garden) and decided this was a fetish I was going to explore no further. Did people really answer classifieds like '*Goody two shoes*? No! Gooey TV shoes! Jenny, a fun-loving TV, would like to meet other tarty TVs for pie-throwing, panty-filling, stockinged-foot squelching slapstick'? Wasn't being a transvestite hard enough without being a tranny who gets her kicks from spreading Angel Delight across her slingbacks?

There was a peepshow a few doors away from the pub.

Ben wouldn't come in with me as he said, being single again, it was not the sort of image he wanted to put across on Old Compton Street. I ignored the quizzical looks of the man on the door and went in. The place looked like a firetrap, but the Licensing Officer had informed me that the easiest way to close down any of these places was on a breach of fire regulations. So it was in the owners' interests to make sure that these came up to standard. I hoped.

There were a number of cubicles, not unlike a polling booth. I went into one which stank of disinfectant and tried not to think about the contents of the tissues scattered across the floor. But at least some customers *had* used tissues because, as I became accustomed to the light, it became clear that most of the customers saw the cubicle walls as a suitable resting place for their ejaculate. I put a pound in a slot and a hole the size of a letterbox flew open.

Inside, there was a woman dressed in a leopard-skin swimming costume. I couldn't guess her age exactly but I knew that my hairdresser would be only too happy to give her a half-price rinse and a Toni. Muzak blared and the game old dear danced away. No, that's not quite true. She staggered for a bit and then headed back to an unmade bed in the corner of the room which was surrounded by crossword books and more used tissues. Then the shutter came down. From what I'd learnt with the Licensing Officer, I knew I'd have to put £6 in the slot for long enough to see her breasts and £9 if the cossie was going to come all the way off. For another £20 and a quick chat with the doorman, oral relief and more can be provided too. I left the peep-show having learned something new. You can teach your grandmother to suck eggs. And then some.

Outside, Ben wanted to know why the voyeur didn't wait until somebody else put £6 in the slot and then put a pound in, so he could join in the action at the point where the dancer already had her breasts out. I was more interested in knowing how the old girl in the leopard skin could possibly manage to get out of her swimming costume unaided in less than three minutes.

Our next stop was the Astral cinema in Brewer Street. There were two films showing – one gay and one straight. We went in and, after an altercation with the doorman, came out again as we'd gone into the men-only 'Gay Men and Safe Sex' entrance and needed the heterosexual *Sun Bunnies* entrance next door. The front-of-house manager in the other cinema seemed just as reluctant to let us in. I asked him what time the next showing of *Sun Bunnies* started.

'The films are continuous,' he said, sounding bored.

'So you can walk in at any time?'

'Yeah, but I wouldn't waste your money. They're only softcore.'

Did Ben and I look like connoisseurs of hardcore? Maybe it was the copy of *Splosh* hanging out of my handbag.

Choosing to heed his warning, we didn't go in but went instead to The Soho Cinema which was a pound cheaper and boasted air-conditioning. 'The Best Sex Films in Soho' it said on the marquee and, tonight, they were showing *Sitting Pretty* and *The Chauffeur*.

The cinema, if you could call it that, as it was more like a wardrobe with a built-in video projection screen, was half full with the same type of men we had seen in the sex shops, only now they had taken off their rain-coats and had them across their laps. I was the only woman there and, as we sat down, the man next to me got up and moved to the end of the row. Soon after, another man came and sat next to me and grunted and fiddled throughout the film, which bore no resemblance to either of the titles listed outside. There were no cars in it and, although the woman on screen was sitting on top of her squash instructor, she couldn't have been described as pretty.

She must have been the only actress in America not to have had her teeth capped or breasts lifted. The sound was appalling but I didn't mind as it meant I didn't have to listen to the dire dialogue. Anyway, I got the gist of what was happening as soon as she dropped her racquet. The film had received the attentions of the censor's pencil and there was nothing remotely salacious about what was left. All come-on and no come. The next scene showed two women *Splosh* fans rubbing liver over each other's breasts. It was clear that one of these women had undergone augmentation. Just like Mickey Mouse's ears, no matter what angle her breasts were at, they remained perfect globes.

Although I expected the audience to be playing with themselves, I didn't expect them to be doing it in pairs. There was a constant toing and froing as the audience swapped seats to try out their luck with the latest arrivals. Ben explained to me that most of the men in the cinema were nominally straight and probably married. I'm sure they thought it was very odd that Ben had chosen to bring his wife with him.

Every couple of minutes or so, somebody would get up and go to the toilet. I made Ben follow one man in and turned my attention back to the film for a scene where a fully dressed woman was led to a sofa by two fully dressed men which ended abruptly before any of them even had a chance to plump a cushion. Ben came back to report that there was a man masturbating at the urinals. Ben had been so embarrassed about disturbing him, he washed his hands to make it look as if there was a reason for him being in there.

'But I think that probably made it look worse,' he said.

In its favour, the Soho Cinema is one of the only picture houses in London which allows you to smoke in the auditorium, but unless you're interested in being jerked off under a Pacamac, its charms wear thin pretty quickly. Although Ben was keen to see if the woman with the breast-lift finally got around to picking the offal up off the lino, we left as we wanted to go to the Festival of Erotica next door. We were a little bit early for the late show, so I showed Ben a clip-joint I'd visited with the Licensing Officer, though there was no way I was going in unaccompanied by an official.

There are around ten clip-joints in Soho (also called hostess bars or near-beer bars) which promise both alcohol and sex and deliver neither. The one I had been into was a small room decorated with fake-brick wallpaper and a few desolate fairy lights. There were two women acting as hostesses and a third pouring drinks from a bar behind a hole in the wall. For one of her special cocktails the price was £109 whereas a glass of non-alcoholic champagne cost a mere £50. If one of the two girls sat with you while you drank it, the cost was another £35. The most shocking thing about these places is that they are completely legal.

Only one customer or a group of friends are allowed in at a time. As far as I could see, the prices were clear enough on the plastic menu, but the thought of sex must do something to these men's brains. They are extremely surprised when they get their bill for £300 or £400 and they haven't even been touched. But it's not a problem if they haven't got the cash on them.

If they are carrying a cash card, they are marched by some heavies, who have appeared from nowhere, to draw out money from a cashpoint machine. If they haven't got this, they are persuaded to sign a promissary note. Many of the customers are married and are frightened of being discovered. Even if they decide to go to the police, it is their word against the owner which is why only one person or a group of friends are allowed in at any one time.

Noting that the woman on the door of the clip-joint was the same 'old dog' (as the Licensing Officer had poetically described her) who had been there on my last visit, we returned to the Revue Bar. The Festival of Erotica, said the posters, had been running for twenty-nine sensational years and I don't think the décor has changed much in that time. I expected Ronnie or Reggie to come through the door with a starlet on their arm any minute. Ben was in raptures as we made our way into the red-velvet lobby.

'I bet it was just like this,' he said stroking the walls, 'when my mum and dad went to see Peters and Lee at the Talk of the Town.'

The show cost £17.50 and, at the Soho going rate, I expected to see one full frontal and the top of another woman's bikini-line. The auditorium was filled with Japanese businessmen plus a few couples who probably knew all the words to 'Welcome Home' too.

A gravelly voice (the same one, I think, that does the warning to look after your handbag in the cinema so that the snake doesn't steal it) came over the sound system to announce the upcoming entertainment and invite the audience to get their drinks from the bar. Ben went to the bar where he was served by the type of woman who calls everyone 'doll' and who hasn't taken off her mascara since the Festival of Britain. The lights went out and, with only seconds to go, Ben reappeared at the front of the auditorium and danced his way up the aisle, convincing most of the Japanese contingent that he was part of the floor show.

There was a fanfare and the silver ruched curtains flew up to reveal nine semi-clad women. As their erogenous zones were already fully on show, I wondered where the performance would go from there. The answer soon became clear – nowhere. After a bit of Tiller Girl type hoofing, the curtain went down again only to rise almost immediately to show that a giant American football helmet had been placed centre stage. One of the dancers, now dressed as a footballer, shimmied around it for a while, then took her clothes off. She finished her act by making enthusiastic love to the helmet and the curtains plummeted again.

That was the general pattern of the show: outsize object centre stage with dancer in front of it dressed in an appropriate outfit, minus the underwear. Thus, we had the Cobra Princess, in snakeskin boots, dance around a big snake and finish with the tail between her legs; Goldie Sparkle who appeared from inside an outsize safe and played seductively with some bullion; and Cherry Thunder, I think that was her name, spinning around on an anti-aircraft gun and ripping off her combat trousers to show us her Victoria Cross.

There was a brief lesbian interlude on 'The Shanghai Express' (the train here represented by a bunk-bed and some sound effects), with two women doing a non-contact top bunk bunk-up. The women were all very glamorous with false eyelashes capable of sweeping the front four rows without their owners leaving the stage. Ben was in Wig Heaven and clapping louder than any of the Japanese, most of whom kept drifting off to sleep due to jet lag. All of the men in the audience had adhered to the Soho dress code and had their raincoats in their laps but I doubt if any of them saw enough to raise even their expectations.

After three women danced around an outsize head of Tutankhamen, which Sphinx-like was losing some of its nose, on came Miss Sugar Cane with her pastry upset. For the finale, all of the girls came back on stage for some more formation dancing.

'Fabulous!' said Ben when the silver curtain came down for the last time. 'Those women were professionals. Not every woman can balance a turban, do nude high kicks and still keep her cervix out of the spotlight.'

The show had lasted an hour and Ben felt it was a quality night out. The Japanese who were still awake did too, while the married couples argued its merit against Peters and Lee all the way back to Theydon Bois. As we left, we passed the barmaid putting on her overcoat.

'See ya doll!' she said to Ben and sucked in deeply on her JPS.

Chapter 16

OL' ONE EYE
IS BACK

Dominic was a bit peeved when I went on my honeymoon with Ben instead of him.

The wedding had gone well but it was odd to be at a party where people expected me to keep my dress on. Actually, halfway through the reception I changed into the rubber dress, almost through habit really. People were quite shocked and it made me realise how far away from the mainstream I'd moved. Fortunately, my mother had already downed the best part of a bottle of champagne at the wedding breakfast so she was oblivious to it. Thankfully she was also totally out of it when Ben took away her handbag and gave her Doris to hold on to instead. It came out lovely in the photographs.

We were too busy to go away on a proper honeymoon but a couple of days after the wedding I did get to spend the afternoon nude in a Kent field with Ben and Pete from the Ring of Confidentes which is more of a honeymoon than a lot of people get.

'Eureka . . . a discovery awaits you. Eureka . . . a revelation in the heart of Kent. Eureka . . . escape and enter the garden of England. Eureka . . . the place you will not want to leave.' The club brochure read like an extract from *Lost Horizons*. I'd been planning to go anyway, after the tip-off in the sauna at Rio's, and I knew that if something other than body painting and nude *It's A Knockout* (two of the club's annual highlights) was happening there, Pete would be able to sniff it out. According to the brochure there were 'numerous well-trodden and less well-trodden paths through the woods in which squirrels, pheasant and less common birds can be seen'. But Pete assured me that there would also be some very common birds in the woods.

Not that the brochure admitted to any impropriety. Running for twenty-seven years the club saw itself as an innocent haven for sun lovers. 'Membership is open to all – families, couples, children and singles – all are united in one thing, a desire to be sociable and naked in the mixed and happy setting that Eureka offers.'

Women were admitted free which I knew meant, 'If we asked the ladies to pay we'd have even less of them here than we have already.' Knowing that the ratio of ball to breast would be roughly ten to one, I hoped that there was a strict enforcement of the club's only rule, 'Thou shalt not annoy'.

Ben and I were having trouble playing the happy couple that afternoon. We had had a row in the morning as Ben said that it was all right for me as I was married now, but pretending to be my other half was doing nothing for his love life. I had to look at his sour face all the way down to Kent on the train and it was all I could do to stop myself throwing my BR coffee at him. When Pete picked us up from the station, I got into the back of the car and Ben took the front seat. It was going to be a war of attrition. After half an hour of Pete focusing his attention on Ben, I was sure Ben would be begging me to be nice to him again, to give him an ally. Initially, Ben seemed to be handling Pete's inquisition quite well. But we would see . . .

'Brace yourself for your first willy,' said Pete as we swung round a bend and into the car-park. And sure enough, there was one, albeit a very small one, emerging from a hatchback with its owner in tow. Pete took us to the clubhouse, where there were five naked men who would never see fifty, or their feet, again. One was the owner, Mark. Pete had warned us that he would try the hard sell and get us to buy an annual membership instead of a day pass. Looking around at the other members, I thought that, at their age, buying an annual pass showed incredible optimism. But Mark merely kissed my hand and pre-empted my thoughts by telling me how unattractive he was. I maintained good eye contact throughout; there was nowhere else safe to look.

We went back outside. Unexpectedly, but thankfully, Pete didn't strip off straight away. Although nudity isn't compulsory at Eureka, I did feel uncomfortable sitting fully dressed in a field surrounded by naked people. Pete didn't help. He started up his sexual inquisition again. The general pattern was something like:

PETE: 'What's the most outrageous thing you two have ever done?'
BEN: 'We quickly normalise all of our experiences. So nothing ever seems outrageous.'

Churlishly, I had to admit that Ben could be evasive for England, such was his skill at deflection.

Pete asked if we thought that there was anything odd about the house in which the Ring of Confidentes party had been held. Aside from the buffet and the occupants, I couldn't think of anything.

'It's a brothel,' beamed Pete.

'I thought some of the women who arrived later on looked like prostitutes,' said Ben, in all seriousness.

Pete looked a bit annoyed. 'They weren't prostitutes.'

However, Samantha with the overheating engine did run her 'massage' business from that address.

'Bit of a busman's holiday for her then,' said Ben. 'You think she'd play golf or something.'

The interrogation went on. Did we like SM? Did I like girls? Were we into piercing? This last question was occasioned by the appearance of a couple, both naked save for their body jewellery. She had pierced nipples while he was wearing a cock-ring. Naturists constantly deny that naturism has anything to do with sex. Yet many of them do things to draw specific attention to the bits they've uncovered. A cock-ring doesn't say 'I'm happy to be at one with nature', it says 'Look what's swinging down there'. Likewise, do nipple rings say 'I am a sun-worshipper', or 'I like having my tits played with'? Another thing. The days of oblong wedge had long since passed. I'm sure that if you put all the nudists in the country in a field, I doubt if you'd find enough pubic hair to make a wig.

The moment of reckoning came.

'Let's go back to the car and strip off,' said Pete.

Undressing in a car-park came second nature to Ben and he was nude in an instant. I kept my knickers on, partly to make Ben look stupid and partly because Pete was already leering at my crotch. When Pete had uncovered ol' one eye, he rummaged in his boot and brought out a chain.

'Do you like the look of this?' he asked, tying the chain around his scrotum.

A couple of inches tighter and I would do. 'It's lovely.'

'I also like to hang things off this,' he said, jamming a finger through a hole in his foreskin. Pete had said earlier that he didn't like piercings so I couldn't work out how the hole got there. Maybe Mrs Pete used it for recorder practice.

Pete led the way out of the car-park. I noticed that Ben was overcompensating for his nakedness by adopting a very jaunty 'look at me' walk. Walking behind him and looking at his bum, I delighted in the discovery that men do get cellulite. Ben turned around to look at me and, for the first time, registered the fact that not only was I still wearing my underwear, I had also taken the added precaution of clutching a bath towel to my bosom.

Sitting under a tree, Pete explained the etiquette for outdoor sex. A couple would go off to the woods and if they were interested in being watched, would look around and indicate to others that they wished to be followed.

'You've got to be a bit discreet, though,' he warned. 'Sometimes the whole field will empty and the couple will be surrounded by dirty old men wanking off.'

I was amazed that Pete believed somehow he fell outside the DOM category. He had explained that Mrs Pete no longer took part in swinging activities having lost her figure, followed swiftly by her confidence. So I took it that his trips to the camp were unaccompanied. Why did he think that when he was having a Jodrell spying on some couple rutting in the shrubbery that he had more integrity?

When Pete decided it was time for us to go into the woods, I wasn't quite sure what the set up was meant to be. Did he think that Ben and I were going to do it in front of him? The only thing Ben and I were prepared to do like a couple was row. Or was he going to find himself a partner and do it in front of us? Were we just there to watch others do it? Did this mean we were expected to jack off in the bracken? And more to the point, jill-off?

Before going into the trees, Pete took us on a quick recce of the camp's lower field known hilariously as The Bottom Field. As with everywhere else in the camp most of the bottoms in the field were over forty, feeling the force of gravity and belonging to men. There were a few younger more attractive rumps but they had gay written all over them. Ben had spotted them and I knew he was seething at having to play Mr Kitty.

What a gentleman Pete was in the woods. Helping me over logs, holding branches out of my way, steering me in the right direction. Only the meanest of hearts would suggest that he was only doing those things in a pathetic attempt to cover up the fact that he was copping a feel. He *was* only doing those things to cover up the fact that he was copping a feel and it was pathetic. There weren't many couples at it in the undergrowth. In fact there weren't any. There were, however, three fully clothed builders installing a cesspit. I passed them by, tensing as I waited for the inevitable catcall. But they were silent. I should have realised. I already had my tits out for the lads.

Pete was like a pig sniffing for truffles. He spotted something glinting in a clearing and bounded off to check it out. Seconds later he was back, breathless.

'Do you want to see a man playing with himself?' he gasped.

Gambling that it wasn't going to be him, I said yes. We moved to a discreet position beside the clearing. The face of the man performing was obscured by a branch but his penis left a lasting impression as it was a dead ringer for Pinhead from the *Hellraiser* films. The shaft was pierced with a series of silver rods, while the head was studded with more rings than the Olympic flag. His performance was, let us say, musical. With him as percussion and Pete as the wind section, we only needed to find a penis that looked like a cello to have a full orchestra.

We moved off again. At various points along the trail, there were trees marked with graffiti saying 'Couples here at . . .' and then giving a time. I thought it may have been wishful thinking on the author's part but Pete insisted that, any minute now, the woods were going to come alive. And to illustrate his point, there was a rustle in the ferns. Pete checked it out.

'Only a couple of queers,' he said to Ben, man-to-man.

Ben looked as if he could just spit. I laughed.

Pete wasn't about to give up. He led us to a fallen tree which, according to him, was a popular site for couples and he suggested we wait around a while. 'You're making my dick twitch,' Pete said to me, pointing to his vibrating member.

I looked as if I could just spit. Ben laughed.

I hugged the towel tighter to my breasts and lit a cigarette. Where were the pheasants and squirrels? There was an uncomfortable silence. No, that's not quite true. The silence was marginally less uncomfortable than actually talking to Pete or Ben. An octogenarian, nude save for his sun-hat, came and joined us on the log. His face was covered in suntan lotion that, for some reason, he had chosen not to rub in. He looked at us and said nothing. As innocent as ever, I thought he was just sitting there giving his pacemaker a break, but after we moved on Pete said, 'What a prick. He was so unsubtle, sat there waiting for us to do something. He could have kept his distance.'

This was uncanny because I had had exactly the same thought in my head about Pete. To prove how subtle he was, he then grabbed me by the waist and asked me what we were going to do now. I squealed and pulled myself away from him.

'Nothing,' I said, with an incredible finality.

Pete wasn't put off. He was seeing me as a challenge. All he felt he had to do was point at his semi-erection enough times and eventually I would keel over and spread my legs. Ben was enjoying my discomfort. Every now and then he would manoeuvre himself between me and Pete to temporarily stop the groping but, as soon as I was starting to feel safe, he would move out of the way and Pete would start all over again.

After one such incident, Pete asked as he moved in on me, 'What does Ben think about men? Does he like them?'

What a depth of perception Pete possessed. 'He doesn't mind.'

'What about threesomes?'

Ben would rather drink muddy water than have you as one point on the eternal triangle. And I'd rather lie

down and sleep in a hollow log than have him. 'I'm not
too sure.'

'I don't mean in the physical sense.'

What on earth was this man on about?

'If you and Ben want to put on a little show, feel free.
I'll be the first to watch.' A little show? Hadn't he
noticed that we were already putting on a first-rate
performance of *Who's Afraid of Virginia Woolf*?

'I've got a really bad headache,' I said, not even both-
ering to waste a good excuse as the man obviously had a
hide like a rhino.

We came out of the woods and my sense of relief was
almost palpable. Pete showed us the swimming-pool and
even though the water was only a couple of degrees
above freezing and the colour of tea, Ben dived in to
avoid any further involvement with Pete or me. I was
livid that he had left me alone again with Pete, but I
later found out that he picked up an eye infection from
the water, which appealed to my sense of justice.

As Ben splashed about in the effluence, I noticed the
couple with the piercings. They were paying us a great
deal of attention. Pete was beside himself.

'Just give it a few minutes. They'll go off and we can
follow them.'

My imaginary headache suddenly became very real. 'I
think that one of my migraines might be coming on.'

Ben emerged from the pool shivering and with his
eyes streaming. He mouthed 'enough' at me as he went
off to towel himself dry.

We followed Ben back to the main lawn and sat down.
Pete wouldn't sit still. He spotted a newly arrived couple
who were young and, in relation to the woofers already
there, very attractive.

'They'll be off in the woods in a minute,' he said. 'They'll give us the nod.'

I lay down on the grass in despair, shutting my eyes as I could see directly between the legs of a woman who was working on her inner labia tan. The afternoon had been one more fantasy dashed. I quite liked the idea of impromptu lovemaking in a field given a frisson by the thought that a farm-hand may be watching from behind a haystack. But being spied on by a group of bollock-naked Chelsea Pensioners?

'You're such a liberated woman,' piped up Pete. 'If I was a woman I'd want to be just like you. How did you get like that?'

'Drink,' offered Ben.

It was incredible. Here I was, in the middle of a nudist camp, showing not so much as an aureole, declining to answer even the vaguest questions about sex and letting all Pete's innuendoes slide over my head. I had done nothing to suggest that I was sexually emancipated in the slightest.

'I'm going to have to go home,' I said. 'It's getting worse.'

Pete had one last look around. 'It's a shame. It's all going to start happening soon . . .'

Back at the car, I was dressed in seconds. Pete was reluctant to put his underpants on and made one final attempt.

'Would you like me to put on a little show for you?'

'Look, she's feeling really ill,' said Ben, finally coming to my rescue. 'I was only joking,' said Pete.

How we all laughed!

Chapter 17

BOTTOM
OF
THE CLASS

I'd almost forgotten that I'd agreed to attend a day school at the Muir Reform Academy. Although the day's events were a foregone conclusion, i.e. I'd get hit a lot, I wanted to see what the other pupils made of it. The night before, I feverishly ironed name tags into all of my clothes, determined that I would do everything to avoid punishment. I had found the proper knee-length socks in Woolworths, but I was still short of the navy blue knickers so I settled for my swinger-proof black roll-on. If it was coming down, it wasn't coming down without a fight.

Although Miss Prim had generously offered to rearrange Ben's interview, he declined, and was therefore unable to attend the day school. To make it up to me, he promised to take me out to dinner afterwards and warned me not to ask the dinner ladies for seconds.

The Academy had relocated for the day to a penthouse

flat in a Bedford tower block. I arrived there and, as instructed, rang the intercom and asked for a 'Mrs Smith'. This turned out to be Gladys, a rotund fifty-five-year-old who showed me into her fluffy pink bedroom, where I changed into my uniform.

'Am I the only girl today?' I asked Gladys, thinking if there were any other women here, I wouldn't sit next to them as they'd have to be completely demented to come to the Academy of their own accord.

'Oh, no,' said Gladys, showing me onto the roof terrace where two other pupils were standing, 'Marjorie'll be coming along soon.'

Just after her medication kicks in, I thought.

Only two other pupils had arrived before me. Dennis was sporting the full Muir Academy uniform of grey flannel shorts, long grey socks, the school tie and a blazer with a badge showing the Academy's emblem of two canes crossing the initials MA. All very authentically schoolboyish if you ignored the fact that Dennis was over seventy and had varicose veins the size of ship's rope. The other pupil was Chris, an attractive, self-employed businessman in his early thirties. His uniform was the same as Dennis's with the addition of a school cap, worn at a rakish angle, and a snake belt. As I came on to the terrace, he was aiming his catapult at the tenants on the balcony of the neighbouring block. I was so embarrassed. I wanted to shout over to the other block and tell them we were council-employed actors doing a community performance of *Blue Remembered Hills*.

Conversation with Dennis and Chris was initially stilted until Chris warmed up, recounting the fabulous times he had spent at the school over the last three years.

'Hastings was brilliant,' he said. 'I really learnt a lot about William the Conqueror and the Battle.'

He explained that there had been some problems with the Hastings venue. It was in the middle of a residential close and the pupils had to sneak around so as not to scare the neighbours. This hadn't prevented them from all going, fully dressed in their uniforms, on a nature ramble in the woods. I hoped Miss Prim wouldn't suggest a repeat of the experience. I would have to tell her I couldn't go because Ben had taken my flower press.

Mark arrived next and I was relieved to see that, like me, he wasn't wearing a blazer. He was a balding, middle-aged chartered accountant who had only been to one proper schoolday before. He would've liked to have come more but his wife was totally unaware of his activities and, as Miss Prim usually left a mark, could only come when his wife and children were away on holiday. Mark was followed soon after by Peter, a plump civil servant who arrived sweating and panting, having run all the way from the train station. These men had travelled from as far afield as Manchester and Yorkshire to attend the school.

My worries about what type of woman Marjorie would be were allayed as soon as I clapped eyes on her. Marjorie was blonde, around forty-five years old, wearing a Burberry skirt, black stockings and a white blouse who told me that she had been in Miss Prim's office typing on the day of my interview. Why was I not worried? Well, you would have had to have been a one-eyed bat with a cataract not to have known that Marjorie was a 'special girl'.

The arrival of Matron caused something of a stir with

Chris and Dennis, the memory of her last assault on their persons still fresh in their minds. Matron was in her late forties with a curly perm and a deep suntan. She was wearing a blue nurse's uniform, unbuttoned enough to reveal an ample cleavage and short enough to show off her stocking tops. Dennis smirked and nick-named her Mrs Squires. I thought he meant Dorothy Squires but apparently he was referring to Squeers in *Nicholas Nickleby*. My failure to retain even the most basic Eng. Lit. facts boded ill.

Gladys was playing school housekeeper for the day. She came out to talk to us while Matron and Miss Prim got the classroom ready. Gladys was game for anything.

'Nothing shocks me,' she said. 'A few weeks ago I rented out the flat to a film company that was making a blue movie. I had a lovely day, sitting here with a bottle of wine watching them.'

This didn't totally surprise me as, when I had been changing in her bedroom, I had noticed a whole stash of porno tapes slipping out from under her bed.

Assembly 10.00 AM
We were summoned in by the bell.

Gladys's lounge had been turned into a classroom with six desks, a blackboard and The Rod Rack. Luckily, in transporting the schoolroom from Hereford, they had forgotten the birch, but in its place was a tawse called 'Black Adder'. Instinctively, I aimed for a seat at the back. It wasn't to be.

'Churchill!' shouted Miss Prim. 'Get to the front now where I can see you.'

Miss Prim then gave me a letter addressed to Ben, the contents of which made the rest of the day a lot easier to bear. After reading Gillian The Punctuator's account of SM pony activities, I had made a few enquiries and written off, in Ben's name, to The Other Pony Club advertised in the Forum Newsletter, saying that he was itching to get down on all fours. I hadn't received any reply but Miss Prim's letter changed that. What a small world it was. It turned out that The Other Pony Club was organised by none other than Miss Prim's consort, Sir Guy Masterleigh. And a gymkhana was coming up very soon. My beret would pale beside Ben's bridle.

Miss Prim then read out the school rules. She explained that four demerits equalled six of the best and told us that we had to stand every time she or Matron came in the classroom. We stood to sing the school hymn. This was an old Shaker song sung very slowly to the tune of Lord of the Dance. Waiting for the first bolt of lightning to hit, I launched into it. The first verse went:

Tis the gift to be simple
Tis the gift to be free
Tis the gift to come down where you ought to be.
And when we find ourselves in the place just right
Twill be in the valley of love and delight.

When we finished, it was time for uniform inspection. My unlawful knickers were skirted over, but, along with Mark, I was chastised for not having a blazer.

'Why haven't you got a school blazer, Churchill?' boomed Miss Prim.

I went for the sympathy vote. 'Because my parents can't afford one, Miss.'

'A charity case are you? Well, you still have to be punished.'

It was probably the same with scholarship kids all over the country. Oh, the iniquities of the class system.

Mark and I had to stand in front of the class and take turns in bending over a chair while Miss Prim gave us six slaps with a paddle. As had happened at the interview, we had to count each one and thank her for the correction. We also collected a demerit each. The others looked slightly disappointed that their uniforms were beyond reproach.

Poetry 10.30 AM
Miss Prim read out two poems, one about a Mr Nobody and the other about a child who would be nice to her mother if their roles were reversed. Our task was then to write a poem on either subject. I knocked off an appalling piece of doggerel which scored five out of ten. Most of the others got the same so there was no punishment. Only Marjorie got full marks and she was awarded a star which was placed on a chart on the wall. I didn't begrudge her that one victory, poor cow, when she'd already lost the battle with her Y chromosomes.

English Language 11.00 AM
We had to write down the reference books for each subject Miss Prim read out. For example, where would you find the definition of a word. Answer – a dictionary. As simple as this may seem, I only got fifteen out of twenty, although I disputed some of the answers. Peter got them all right and the creep proudly put the first of many stars next to his name. Mark, on the other hand, had done appallingly and was called to the front.

'What happens when you come last?' asked Miss Prim.

'Last in the class gets six of the best!' we all chorused.

Dennis was fidgeting. Miss Prim told him to stop but he wouldn't. Called to the front, he was given a hard slap on the back of his legs which couldn't have done his varicose veins any good. Thick green and blue threads pulsed angrily across his calves. Bellicose veins, I thought, biting my nails. Miss Prim saw me doing it and gave me another demerit. It seemed a piffling crime but then I suppose the whole object of the exercise was to be punished.

Maths 11.30 AM
What chance did I have against a chartered accountant? Actually, Mark didn't do that well but I came bottom in percentages with twelve out of twenty-seven. Peter got another star which I, beginning to get into the role, peeled off as I bent over to take my punishment.

'Last in the class gets six of the best!' shouted the boys and Marjorie, eager no doubt to see my roll-on pulled down.

Miss Prim didn't oblige, merely lifting my skirt. She commented on my non-regulation knickers.

'They were dyed in the wash, Miss,' I said, as her hand came down.

Break 12.00 noon
Gladys brought out coffee and the kind of E-number laden snacks favoured by hyperactive children. They were revolting and I sneaked off for a cigarette even though tobacco was banned. I wasn't caught, but Chris was punished for stealing a carrot magnet off Gladys's fridge.

Latin 12.15 PM

The only Latin I know is *coitus à mamilla*. I had taken the metalwork option at school, so I asked Miss Prim for a special dispensation. My plea fell on deaf ears. Dennis squirted me with his water pistol. I was going to retaliate by shouting the words 'Nursing Home' at him but Miss Prim obviously had eyes in the back of her head as she whirled around from the blackboard and caught him red-handed.

'Out here, you horrible little boy!' she growled. 'I'm going to get Matron to deal with you.'

Matron was beside herself. Stern but excited, she pulled down Dennis's shorts and pants, bent him over her lap and gave him a sound walloping with her hand.

We had to give the definition of Latin words and, amazingly, I managed to get all but one right. Peter got another star. Mark, bottom again, was given a thrashing on his bare bum with a Victorian malacca cane. At this stage I was wondering what the sexual element was for these men and Marjorie. I sneaked a peek at their crotches while they were being spanked to see if they were sporting erections. Nothing. Although I'm sure there was the beginning of a bulge when Dennis was seen to by Matron but it was probably just another vein.

Our lessons were interrupted by the sudden appearance of the block caretaker on the roof terrace. We were told to keep quiet until she was gone. (Gladys later told me a little bit about the caretaker. 'She's on a meat-free diet, that one,' she said. I told Gladys that I didn't understand why the caretaker's vegetarianism was worthy of a mention. 'No, she's a lesbian,' said Gladys.) Miss Prim instructed the boys to take off their ties and roll down their socks when they went to lunch so as not to bring undue attention to themselves. What Marjorie was meant to do was anybody's guess. I didn't think the care-taker would have been fooled either. Unless she mistook them for Morris dancers.

Art 12.45 PM
We were given a drawing of a Victorian schoolroom to colour in. While we were doing this, Miss Prim gave us a brief history of a Victorian school and the various ways in which discipline was maintained. The boys cooed in awe. I coloured most of my picture in brown on the grounds that I didn't think that there was that much colour in a Victorian schoolroom. I was bored and glad when it was time for lunch.

Lunch 1.15 PM
'Line up behind each other. Six inches apart between the boys and girls,' commanded Miss Prim.

We lined up outside the kitchen for our packed lunches. Chris, who by this time had gone into total regression, was shouting about how smelly girls were. I gave him a swift punch to the kidney which shut him up and then kicked him in the shins to drive the point home. Matron watched on approvingly.

I didn't have any problem saving myself for Ben's treat as, for lunch, Gladys provided cheese spread sandwiches, a yoghurt and another batch of her nightmare snack food. The conversation was strange. Sometimes we kept in character, teasing each other over the lessons (Chris was jumping around, waving his cap and scaring the neighbours again), and then we would slip into our grown up personas. Mark explained that part of the attraction of the school was giving up adult responsibility.

He found being in management extremely stressful and coming to Miss Prim for a day got rid of all the tension. It was the same story with everybody. Nobody admitted to being turned on by coming to the Academy – everybody was merely there to relieve stress. Hadn't any of them heard of a Newton's cradle? Far from relieving my stress, I felt that the day's events so far had probably doubled my blood pressure level. It was only the thought of seeing Ben getting his oats (literally) that was keeping me going.

Lunch eaten, I sneaked off to smoke behind a plant pot. No sooner had I lit up, than Miss Prim was leaning over me, demanding to know what I was doing.

'You know you're not allowed to smoke, Churchill, especially without permission. That's twelve of the cane for you after lunch and another demerit.'

Peter hadn't seen me reprimanded and when he started smoking, I kept silent so that Miss Prim would catch him too. She did.

After lunch, I argued that my punishment was unfair as I had not been informed of this rule and probably wouldn't have smoked at all. Or rather, I would have made a much better job of not being caught. I still had to have the twelve strokes. It was agony. Unlike the other instruments, the cane concentrates the pain in a specific area. I struggled to get out of her grasp.

'Matron,' called out Miss Prim, 'Come in here and hold this girl down.'

Matron wedged my head in her bosom and held me tight. I considered using the safe word, 'pax', but I knew if I did, I would be out of the game.

Miss Prim showed no sympathy. 'Perhaps if you had the regulation knickers on, Churchill, it wouldn't have been so painful.'

I didn't believe her.

'I'm surprised that you've been so naughty,' said Matron, smoothing down her skirt. 'Girls are normally so much better behaved than boys.'

I'm going to have Ben horseshoed, I thought as I went back to my seat.

Art (cont.) 2.00 PM

Sore, I returned to colouring in my drawing. I was rudely interrupted by a plastic scorpion landing in my lap. The culprit was Dennis. He had also stolen Peter's exercise book and Mark's ruler. Miss Prim selected a new cane from the many she had at her disposal and Dennis's trousers came down again As he bent over Miss Prim's desk, I reminded her that Dennis was meant to get six more for ripping out the pages of his exercise book. All the others started to chant 'grass' at me, but I thought I had probably done Dennis a favour. Marjorie giggled which led to her first punishment. We were denied the opportunity to see what Marjorie had up her kilt, as Miss Prim chastely spanked her over the top of it.

Essay Writing 2.30 PM

Using the drawing, we had to write an essay incorporating parts of the picture, such as the schoolmaster and the children standing at the front of the class. I had now got the hang of what these exercises were about and used our class as the main basis of my essay. My wit was at the level of calling the teacher 'Master Bates'. But Matron and Gladys were called in to listen to it and, at last, I received full marks and a star. Strangely enough, it felt good.

Reading 3.00 PM

We had to read aloud from a storybook aimed at eleven-year-olds. I read out a story about beavers which was as close as we came all day to anything remotely sexual. I was told off for gabbling, but I just wanted it over and done with. I was beginning to feel like a complete prat and couldn't wait for the whole thing to be over so I could go out to dinner with Ben.

Grammar 3.30 PM

An exercise on homonyms was a bit more taxing but I didn't fare too badly. As usual, Peter got a hundred per cent. This time it was Chris's turn to get the six for being last.

General Knowledge 4.00 PM

A test on inventors and their inventions. I came last. I did better on familiar sayings and a general knowledge test. Mark came last. Poor Mark, I thought as he was caned. Then I corrected myself. Lucky Mark, I thought as he was caned.

Form Period 4.30 PM

Miss Prim counted up the demerits we had accumulated. I had three and was, therefore, spared the cane. But I was put on a defaulter's list which meant you had to go into Gladys's bedroom and be knocked around the plush by Miss Prim and Matron in private. Again, I begged ignorance. Miss Prim let me off, but she must have been wondering why I had come.

As each boy, and Marjorie, went into the bedroom, I felt ecstatic that I had escaped this last punishment. The sound of hands against bare flesh reverberated all around the flat. Each pupil, in turn, came out sweating and red-faced. By now, I had my feet up with a cup of coffee, talking to Gladys about what 'normal' was; I had no idea any more. Matron emerged, flushed and victorious, and had to rush off for her train as she had another of her boys visiting that night.

Hometime 5.00 PM

At last we were allowed to change and I could have a cigarette without fear of retribution. Even when Marjorie had changed, he still looked a bit odd as he was wearing shorts which showed off his depilated legs. Chris was back to reminiscing about Hastings and the hazelnut sticks Miss Prim had used on him. At six feet long, they were a force to be reckoned with. It was, said Miss Prim, one of those times when Matron had needed to change her knickers.

Miss Prim took me aside and asked me how I'd enjoyed my day. I told her it was fine aside from the cane. The pain from it was almost unbearable. She commiserated with me and confessed to having a similar problem.

'My husband doesn't know that I can take the birch endlessly. If he used the cane I'd be begging for mercy.' As I said goodbye she promised to show me how much easier the birch was on my next visit.

Embarrassingly, I had to get the train back to London with Peter. I kept the conversation neutral all the way home, feigning a huge interest in the machinations of the civil service. As we parted from each other at King's Cross, Peter told me that the first thing he was going to do when he got home was look at his marks in the mirror. He didn't need to add what he intended to do then.

The whole day had been a big masturbatory fantasy for everyone but me. I was learning the lesson that it was nigh on impossible to step into somebody else's fetish and expect to gain some sexual excitement from it.

This didn't mean Ben was off the hook regarding the Pony Club. Far from it, as his choice of restaurant for dinner that evening sealed his fate with the saddle once and for all. For Ben took great delight in booking a table for three (Dominic wanted to see my face too, when I found out where I was being taken) at yes, School Dinners, the sexy schoolgirl theme restaurant. There was some small consolation when, at the end of the evening, after spending £150, Ben said, 'I could have got a deeper sexy-schoolgirl charge from buying a geometry set'.

We were ushered into the restaurant by the doorman who told us to, 'Talk to Clodagh Rogers over there on the till'.

Clodagh, who actually bore a far greater resemblance to Julie Walters, relieved Ben of £80 for the food and sent us to the bar. The place was empty aside from a couple of seedy-looking businessmen and the waitresses who were dressed in standard sexy schoolgirl kit. I was piqued that they had made a better job of it than me, although from the amount of cash they managed to take from us over the course of the evening, Midland Bank blouses would have been more appropriate attire.

On the walls hung photographs of famous past customers – to think, we would be eating in a place frequented by Prince Andrew, Janet Jackson and Freddie Starr! The ceiling was covered in what I assume was meant to be humorous graffiti: 'Women for babies – men for fun', 'Amnesia Rules – O', that kind of thing. I noticed, too, a framed letter from a journalist on the *Chicago Tribune* asking if she could do a piece on the restaurant. I suppose as a signifier of the English at sex, School Dinners was perfect: smutty, filled with innuendo and totally bereft of eroticism.

According to its publicity leaflet, School Dinners is as famous as the Ritz or Harrods (neither of which it bore any resemblance to) and every cab driver in London would know of its location (aside from the one who drove us from Hackney). The restaurant is based on the 1950s *St Trinian's* films and was first opened in 1981. The leaflet said, 'School Dinners is exceptional in that it provides both men and women, aged from eighteen to eighty, with the most enjoyable and memorable evening they are ever likely to experience in a restaurant. Your choice of a three course meal from our superb, comprehensive menu catering to all tastes and preferences, will be served by either our gorgeous stocking-clad schoolgirls, or for the ladies – our muscle-bound schoolboy boarders, all under the supervision of our cane-brandishing, laugh-a-minute headmaster.'

The laugh-a-minute headmaster was the man on the door. His name was Kim and he had no need of the cane as his tongue was a deadly weapon. He was very camp and I didn't understand why he wanted to work in such a heavily heterosexual environment until he explained that he was very, very well paid for dishing out insults to the stag parties and hen nights. As we'd booked late, none of the sexy schoolboys were on duty and, as with everything else, I was going to be the only woman there bar the waitresses. Two stag parties turned up and I found it hard to believe that out there, somewhere, there were two women desperately waiting to marry two of these men.

It could have only been Gladys who wrote the line 'superb comprehensive menu'. We sat at our table, and ordered (wearing plastic bibs), taking in Kim's warning not to go for the pâté as even dogs refused to eat it. Why the dogs singled out only the pâté for their disapproval was anybody's guess as the food was uniformly disgraceful. How a meal could go so wrong in a microwave, I don't know.

Party games followed the meal. First off, a nominated member of each table had to get up and do a turn on the Karaoke. The punishment for bad singing was to be caned by one of the waitresses. I shoved Ben's hand up to volunteer. If I got to see him being hit then the evening wouldn't be a complete loss. When it was his turn, the headmaster passed him over. I asked him why.

'Sisterhood,' said Kim.

Curses.

Musical chairs came next and, while one of the waitresses lined up some chairs, another was fighting off one of the diners who'd groped her. Both Dominic and Ben (or Butch and Bitch as Kim introduced them) had to play. Dominic was out straight away but Ben, ever competitive, was out to win, elbowing one of the grooms off his chair in the process. He needn't have bothered as Kim was fixing it so that he did win by prior arrangement with me. For there could only be one prize. Kim's efforts were nearly foiled when Ben sat on the lap of the last man in but recovered by declaring them joint winners.

One of the sexy schoolgirls was brought out to lightly chastise the other winner but, when it came to Ben, Kim handed the cane over to me. I think the stag parties were a bit taken aback by this mad woman laying into her dining companion with such vehemence. It seemed such a public place for such a private moment.

My revenge didn't end there. As my final act of retribution of the day, I arranged it with Kim for Ben to receive the restaurant's speciality, 'The Kneetrembler'. And so Ben was placed on a chair in the middle of the restaurant with a sexy schoolgirl on his knee, force feeding him trifle with her fingers. Most of the trifle went over his head. The erotic appeal of the evening went over mine. It cost me £15 to see him thus humiliated. When the sexy schoolgirl had finished, she asked Ben to put a tip down the leg of her stockings and didn't take too kindly when he tried to put five pound coins down there.

'Did you enjoy that?' I asked him when he sat down.

'Her fingers smelt of old flannel,' said Ben.

Indeed, she had been wiping down tables only moments earlier.

Chapter 18

LES FESSEURS

Though it's hard to believe, I had another equally sexy dinner out, quite soon after School Dinners, with the members of the Moonglow Dining Club.

They could dress it up any way they wanted to but the club was basically a group of men who liked knocking women around. Its magazine, *The Moonglow Courier*, said, 'The Moonglow Dining Club offers a unique opportunity for enthusiasts to come together to discuss, view and participate in a wide variety of spanking activities. Members include single ladies and gentlemen as well as couples. The action is always strictly gentlemen dominant, ladies submissive.'

The Courier advertised itself as 'essential reading for discerning dominant gentlemen and their compatible companions'. Surprisingly, its editor was a woman, Alison. The first page set the whole tone of the magazine. There was a photograph of a topless tabloid model.

The caption underneath read, 'Is this the look of a girl about to be caned? The lovely young lady apparently pranged her car just before the photoshoot. Now if she knew that there was a furious boyfriend waiting at home, his hand itching to use the cane on her fabulous bottom, is this the look that she would be wearing?' I studied the look and guessed it was the only one she had. Like a broken lock on a toilet door, it would only ever say 'Vacant'.

The magazine carried the results of its readership survey. Only twenty per cent of its readers had filled in the questionnaire. I presumed the rest had wanted to but had left their Biro in their other anorak. The typical reader was outlined as a non-graduate male, in his fifties, managerial in status and, surprise, surprise, living alone. Ten percent of the readers *were* female but none had replied to the survey as it was quite painful to write in traction.

Schoolgirl scenarios were not a comfort to these sad bachelors in their mid-life crises but other uniformed women were. Casual outfits, even sexy ones, were another no go area as were women in their thirties. Said Alison, 'What women in their thirties have done to court disapproval is a mystery, but the preferred ages were overwhelmingly twenties and forties.' Being a woman in her thirties, I know what the problem is. It's a tricky age, post-stupid and pre-senile, when the idea of being beaten up in a Wren's uniform by a war baby without any O levels holds little allure.

I nearly signed up as a Kelly Girl when I read that around thirty per cent of the respondents had spanked their secretary at some time. Two-thirds liked a girl to be lectured before punishment, sixty per cent thought she should be humiliated and half thought attire should be inspected. Impressively, a third of respondents actually lived with women who didn't require inflation before intercourse. Of these men, one hundred per cent claimed to be having extra-marital affairs with enthusiastic partners. These enthusiastic partners probably were inflatable: 'Tip Talking Laura's head forward and she says "yes"'.

Having gleaned a greater understanding of the readership, I moved on to the magazine's fiction section and a story entitled 'MI Six of the Best'. This featured a fictional MI6 training camp located in the remote Cotswold village of Much Beating which specialised in producing female James Bonds. As part of the tough training, the 'young ladies' were subject to a strict disciplinary regime. 'He wasted no time in applying the first stroke; the girl groaned and a red stripe slowly surfaced across what had been a virginally unmarked rump. But the plucky young soldier took it stoically.'

Unable to take too much of it stoically, I turned to the film review section. The film in question was *La Fessée ou Les Memoirs de M. Leon, Maître-Fesseur*. Unfortunately, it was never shown in competition at Cannes and so *The Spanking or The Memoirs of Mr Leon, Master-Spanker* was cruelly denied a crack at the Palme D'Or. To rectify this glaring oversight, the reviewer spent five pages exploring its complex themes, all illustrated with breathtaking stills. As the editor rightly pointed out, the reviewer gave us more than Barry Norman ever did.

Keeping the highbrow tone going was the Philosophical Slot. In this issue the subject was 'Understanding Spanking', a direct lift, I felt, from Descartes. Apparently, for women, 'the sexual excitement is to some a matter of plumbing. Warmth from a well-smacked bottom flows to neighbouring areas, setting off in particular the clitoral area. Thus, purely for physical reasons, the vagina becomes moist and aroused from a spanking. The mechanics of clenching and releasing the bottom cheeks also creates movements in the vagina area. Just rubbing a lady's bottom enthusiastically can bring about an orgasm in many women; try it sometime!' But careful: spank too hard and you have to get the pump out again.

The editorial then went on to explain that the female orgasm also included the brain, therefore a spanking scenario must include a mental build up. There is, it said, 'a superb and most successful reason for administering a spanking to a lady; jealousy, feigned or real. If you spank a lady for flirting, for instance, it will do wonders for her feelings for you. She will think you care deeply and it is surprising what you can get away with.'

After ten pages advertising 'Tools of Transformation' (travel whips for sadists on the move were a popular seller), I came to the contacts section. Some were from women, although it seems that the constant beatings were going to their heads:

> I have been described throughout my life as a very stubborn, wilful, even spoilt, little madam (but all I ever wanted was my own way; really that's not too much to ask, is it?) and have been told that what I need in my life is a strict male authority (possibly even a father figure sometimes) who won't put up with any nonsense nor be afraid to put me over his knee from time to time. (Honestly, I think people who make remarks like these are really horrid!)

They tell me that he must be capable of being very stern when necessary, but as I am quite nice as well really, must also be very kind and caring. If you think that you are this man, I would love to hear from you. I am in my early forties, an attractive, slim brunette and ridiculously young for my age.

And ridiculously old for her IQ.

The magazine seemed to vacillate between being academic (extensively quoting the Danish feminist Maria Marcus on why she enjoyed CP) and being as prurient as the newspapers it criticised in its editorial. Quoting the *Daily Sport*, it related the story of a director of a nursing home who wound up in an industrial tribunal when some teenage girls claimed unfair dismissal. The girls were spanked with a ruler, brush and fish slice as well as the traditional hand. The snippet ended with the *Courier*'s conclusion, 'Perhaps they deserved it!'

The club also sent me a list of forthcoming attractions. They had over 500 members with around 170 actually attending their functions, the rest being content with the club video list. Events were held every six weeks or so, all around the country. At these meetings, around twelve 'gentlemen' would administer to the behinds of half a dozen (paid) 'ladies'. In the offing were the fourth meeting of the Severity School Housemasters in Luton and The Wren's Return in Birmingham which was 'a chance for members to instil some military discipline into some rather attractive recruits'.

In addition, over the coming month, Moonglow was taking its road show to Manchester and London. These road shows were, apparently, ideal for new members to

find out what the club was actually about (as if the
Courier had been loaded with ambiguity) and 'for other
members who mainly like to watch nubile young ladies
have their bottoms thoroughly warmed. All will have
some chance to participate but most of the action will be
carried out by experienced members who can perform
to a very high standard.'

George, the club president, had written saying that, as
I may have guessed, there were five male members for
every female one and consequently, it was important
that the ladies were clear on the level of involvement
they were seeking. I rang him to discuss the matter, saying that I would like to be an observer at the road show,
just to see what it was like. George agreed that this was
an excellent idea because only experienced members
would be participating as sometimes a new guy could get
a little out of hand. He reassured me that he would be
protective of me. I couldn't decide whether to find this
reassuring or not, but I paid my £75.

We were all to meet at an east London tube station
and then George would ferry us to the location at a photographer's studio near by. I didn't bother to ask how I
would identify anybody. I'd know.

At the station, I spotted a man in his early forties with
a face from a sex crime photofit. Dressed all in black and
looking furtive, I knew I had found a fellow Moonie.
Soon after that, two other men appeared, one in his seventies in a linen suit, the other fortyish and sweating
profusely in a tweed jacket. Both looked as though they
expected the dogs to catch up with them at any second.
A fourth man arrived. I watched him go to each of the
men and say the word Moonglow out of the corner of
his mouth. It was George. Nobody spotted me as a

prospective member and, as they stood huddled in a group, I had to jump above their shoulders to introduce myself. They looked shocked. Perhaps they thought I was Juliet Bravo.

George was true to his word about looking after me. He made the three men squeeze into the back of his car so that I could sit in the front. He probably regretted this chivalry later when the weight of them led to his exhaust pipe being smashed on a speed bump. Thankfully, the journey was a short one. George told me that he used to be in the City and was now the MD of a security company. Albert, the septuagenarian, commented excitedly that a road we had passed was called Paradise Row.

The photographer's studio, in Purgatory Alley, was buzzing with activity. I hadn't eaten as the Moonglow was a dining club and my heart sank when I saw a pile of Sainsbury's sandwiches on a table next to a couple of bottles of Lambrusco. What was it with deviant sexuality and bad wine? Fortunately, the screw top was easier than a cork on my shaking fingers and I sat down with a glass and tried to look inconspicuous.

I wasn't alone for long. Leonard, a grandfatherly man with a white handlebar moustache and liver spots, pulled up a rocking chair and asked, 'Were you spanked at home or school?'

'At home,' I replied.

'So you fantasize about being spanked, then?'

In your dreams old man.

'Why are you here? Are you a model?'

'Certainly not.' I'd been around this scene long enough to know a euphemism when I heard one.

Leonard, who seemed quite upset that they had

stopped corporal punishment in schools, had been a member of the Moonglow club since its inception four years earlier. A real spankophile, he had amassed a large collection of books, videos and magazines on the subject. He had even written five spanking limericks for the next issue of the *Courier*. I'd heard that's how Edward Lear got started too.

Other members sat quietly eating their sandwiches or discussing the problems of travelling to the meeting from Leeds and Somerset. The age group was forty upwards and most of them looked relatively normal, but then my judgement of normality wasn't as good as it had been before I started my quest.

Aside from his Moonglow presidency, George was also in the video business. He was talking to Victor, another videomaker, about the bum of one of his starlets. 'How long do you think it will take for the bruises to go?' asked Victor.

'I should think about ten days,' guessed George.

'So if we started filming two weeks after you do, we should be okay.'

George agreed. Damn it was tough working with these method actresses.

As George was discussing his next œuvre (seemingly undaunted about working in the shadow of *La Fessée ou Les Memoirs de M. Leon, Maître-Fesseur*), two young Meryl Streep wannabees arrived with a short, dumpy man who I took to be their manager. They looked about eighteen, were badly dressed, hungry for their turn under the arc lights and, even by Moonglow standards, something of an embarrassment. They were too young for Moonglow tastes (female members have to be over twenty-three and men twenty-six) but declared with a loudness which increased with their consumption of Lambrusco that they were professionals and that one of them had a baby to feed. They were later joined by an older woman who seemed already to have starred in films.

Sandwiches finished, it was time to open the meeting. This was carried out as if we were all at a productivity conference. Then the girls came in. There was Alison (this is just her spanking name), editor of the *Moonglow Courier*, who was a pleasant looking woman in a short, red satin dress, black stockings and stilettos, Then came Sharon, who was dressed in a similar fashion with long black hair and a pouting red mouth; and Rose, who was tall and patrician looking, and dressed in a black lace top with a figure-hugging black mini-skirt. They appeared to be in their mid to late twenties. They sat at the front while George introduced them.

To warm up the proceedings, the girls had to choose a man to give them a spanking. Alison picked Leonard and had to help him up from his rocking chair. Leonard sat on a chair in front of everybody and Alison bent over his lap. He pulled up her dress to reveal a pair of very brief black knickers. He practically drooled.

'Such a creamy white bottom,' he said, remembering the advice given in the *Courier*'s Philosophy slot that a bum had to be admired and rubbed. 'These things have to be taken slowly.'

Too slowly for George who told Sharon to pick another man at the same time. She chose Mr Photofit. His heart didn't seem to be in it and he gave her a few desultory smacks. Rose chose Albert. Albert had to take things easy as well – any great exertion would have probably killed him. As he lightly palmed Rose's rear, the audience commented on the largeness of it. As two of her cheeks wouldn't have made one of mine, I was glad that I hadn't paid to participate. When the three men had finished, the girls claimed to be disappointed that the spanking hadn't been harder.

Then the experienced members took over. In the first scenario, Alison was a naughty eighteen-year-old who had stayed out at a disco beyond curfew. Her guardian, John, was waiting for her when she got in. 'Just what time do you call this, young lady?' asked John, tapping his watch.

'Two-thirty,' replied a sullen Alison.

'I told you to be in at ten-thirty. I promised your parents I would look after you.'

Alison shrugged belligerently.

John was at his wits' end. What would Penelope Leach do in this situation? He knew. He put Alison across his lap, pulled down her knickers and soundly spanked her.

She was unrepentant. 'I was with Leonard,' she said, challenging John's authority, 'and he was so good.'

Leonard was beaming.

The scene finished and we all clapped. The whole thing was then played out again, this time with Ray worrying over the whereabouts of Rose and Sharon. The acting was better and therefore the spanking harder. Ray's preferred method was to hammer on one cheek at a time until it was the colour of claret. It looked as though Rose wouldn't be doing too much film work in the coming week, as Ray's rings had left some deep marks. We applauded again and the girls went off to change for the next skit.

During the break, Victor complained to the older female film star about one of his actresses who had walked off the set in mid-production after fearing her father might find out. He had promised to pay her £300 for five hours work and he was wondering how much he should deduct.

'The problem with these girls,' he said, 'is that they see noughts in front of their eyes and don't think of the consequences. After twenty minutes, a lot of them find that they can't take the pain.'

Still, the film could be saved, he said. They were going to use a bum double.

Victor then turned to me. Having talked about my experience of fetish clubs and the Muir Reform Academy, Victor took me for an old hand, and name-checked every CP fanatic in London. As I knew none of them, I talked more about Miss Prim.

'Schoolgirl videos just walk off the shelves,' said Victor, 'but I won't make them. Too many little school-girls are attacked and I don't want to be associated with pervs like that.'

In the next scene, Alison played a wayward security officer whose boss had found out she'd been slacking on the job. Little was left to my imagination as, directly in front of me, she was forced to bend over a high stool with her Securicor knickers around her ankles. I guessed she wasn't about to have her pay packet docked. As she worked in a footwear factory, it was fit-ting that she be spanked with the sole of a shoe. Quite where the riding crop came into it, I don't know, but I applauded enthusiastically at the end anyway.

It was time for the cautionary tale of the unsuitably dressed secretary played by Sharon. Rose, the severely attired office supervisor, brought this indiscretion to the attention of her boss, George. George took pity on her and presented her with a £50 voucher for Wallis.

Actually, I'm lying, but by now I was feeling that some of the script writing could do with a little tinkering. But hold – this scene had a twist. As Sharon hiked up her non-regulation panties, she let go of a secret. Rose, Little Miss Butter-Wouldn't-Melt, had had her hand in the till. She was summoned to George's office and given an ultimatum – drop your drawers or pick up your P45. Rose kept her job. We clapped, we cheered, we said how lovely their bottoms were now that they were warming up.

Another break. Rose came over and asked if I was interested in doing this type of work. Having just received another extortion letter from my bank manager, I thought hard before saying no. Rose, who was well-spoken and by far the best actress, told me that she was genuinely into the fetish and SM scene and had decided she might just as well make money out of it.

'Are you submissive or dominant?' she asked.

'Mainly submissive but I change roles sometimes.' About as often as I changed the sheets, actually, but I had an idea where the conversation was going.

'I don't like dominating men,' she said. And then a pause for dramatic effect. 'But I do women.'

With that, she was off to climb into her schoolgirl outfit.

As I was thinking that maybe red Lambrusco doesn't taste too bad when you're drinking it to avoid talking to anybody, a man in a 'Stop the Acid Rain' T-shirt came and sat behind me. He obviously felt that shampoo was destroying the planet too as he hadn't washed his hair for a month.

'Somebody come and talk to her,' he said. 'She's all by herself.'

As I turned around to smile in gratitude, he asked, 'Are you a reporter? We all think you are – that's why we're being quiet.'

I covered myself by talking about how I couldn't stand the cane because of the pain and rattled off a list of every CP instrument that Miss Prim had used on me. He was dead impressed.

He was Alison's husband. Now convinced of my CP credentials, he told me some tender love stories about him and Alison. Misty-eyed, he remembered the time that a friend of his spanked Alison in the back of a transit van. Being so love struck, he made his friend rub Ralgex into Alison's raw behind. Being so totally smitten, she hit the roof and had to go sit in a puddle. All the world loves lovers and I felt that my heart had been Ralgexed too, as he told me how they spent their free time walking hand in hand through car-boot sales looking for things he could hit her with. Why, only the other day, they had found a weightlifter's belt!

Leonard joined us, also in a sentimental mood. Were there tears in his eyes as he recalled how, at the Luton Severity School, they had broken a wooden paddle over one woman's tushie? They assured me that no blood was ever spilt, but Alison confessed that her bruising had only just gone down.

'It's not the actual pain,' Alison's husband told me. 'It's the fantasy factor of the whole situation.' I felt reassured. They were only fantasy bruises.

Leonard thought I looked as if I wanted to spank the girls. I assured him I could wait for another time. Better still, some old romantic chipped in, perhaps Leonard could spank me.

Fortunately, the arrival of the schoolgirls stopped this

unscheduled scenario developing. This was the final scene; I felt this time surely the denouement had to be different. There were three headmasters who took turns wearing George's headmaster gown. Alison was in trouble for having an atrocious school report, Sharon for cheating in an exam and Rose for being a bad headgirl. There was the usual lecturing and calls for more discipline. Did George then do an about turn and say that maybe the Montessori approach was right after all? No, he did not. Post caning, we had to inspect each of the girls' bottoms and rank them in order of markings. Sharon came top as hers was the boniest.

George then rose to call the meeting to a close. They finished at five, said George, for those who had to convince their spouses that they had had another hard day at the office. He informed those of us who were planning to stay that there were stroke mags on sale and that the new video release would be delayed because of problems with one scene. Apparently, one of the actresses had regained her sanity for a moment.

The 'manager' of the two young girls asked if anyone was interested in a long weekend of spanking at a country house in France.

'It's the wives that are a problem,' said George.

I couldn't understand why. *The Courier* had said that if you spanked them hard enough you could get away with anything. But at a recent four-day event in Pucklechurch, only Leonard had managed to stay the course.

The sweaty tweed jacket, who had been sitting next to me all afternoon in silence, nodded sadly in agreement to this. His wife thought that he was still working at Heathrow that afternoon. I asked him if he had enjoyed himself. He had and felt it was much better than watching videos. 'Nothing beats live action,' he said smiling and then sweated some more.

George invited us to mix with the girls. As with most of the sexual endeavours I had become involved in over the previous months, what actually happened was less distressing than the tedium it provoked. I couldn't wait to go home. Annalise was working on a difficult eyebrow in *Neighbours*.

Chapter 19

PLEASE LEAVE
THE
DUNGEON TIDY

'It's a lovely little B&B in Cornwall,' said Ben.

I'd been complaining again about not having a honeymoon because of my commitment to other people's sex lives so Ben had looked around for a suitable weekend break for Dominic and me.

'Westward Bound is the perfect romantic environment for being alone with your loved one, in a luxurious and overwhelming environment,' he said, reading from the brochure. 'Oh yes, and it's got a dungeon . . .'

Well, it was as close to two weeks in Torremolinos as I was going to get, so I booked. Westward Bound is run by a couple called Sadi and Steve who also run a fetish clothing company under the same name. Keen to distance themselves from the idea that they run a brothel, there is no personal service, guests have to be over twenty-one and the dungeon is reserved for the sole use of one couple at a time, no groups or singles. What would a person on their own do in a dungeon anyway? Slap themselves stupid?

'The dungeon,' said the brochure, 'measures twenty-five by twenty feet and has been carefully decorated to provide ample scope for the private fantasies of most persons . . . our emphasis is on style and comfort rather than sleaze and tack.' That was important. There was nothing like a sleazy, tacky dungeon to put you off your nipple clamps. Despite the assurance of style and comfort, there was one major drawback to the place. You weren't allowed to smoke there. It must have been on health grounds. After all, it was a terrible thing to do, ruining your lungs when you were flagellating somebody to within an inch of their life.

Dominic was prepared to commit this ultimate act of masochism (though he did suggest wearing nicotine patches) for the chance finally to get away with me. To say he was excited was an understatement. Putting his foot down on the motorway, we didn't even have time to commit that other act of ultimate masochism – stopping for lunch at a Little Chef. I could appreciate his urgency. At £175 for the night, we couldn't afford to miss a moment of torture time. We had arranged to meet Sadi and Steve at a garage and then follow their car to their house. There's money in muck, I thought, as our battered Ford Escort groaned along behind their nearly new Mercedes.

Their 1920s English country house was set in its own grounds, with beautiful views of the surrounding countryside. More importantly, the house could not be overlooked by any locals. Steve seemed quiet and a trifle nervous. Sadi, on the other hand, was a peroxide blonde dominatrix and completely in control. Sadi showed us to

our room and ordered us not to go down to the
dungeon until she came back up.

'Make yourselves comfortable,' she commanded.

If Laura Ashley had been the set designer for
Pasolini's *Salo, 120 Days of Sodom*, she would have come
up with something pretty much the same as Westward
Bound. The pink of the counterpane on the bed
matched the pink of the curtains and it was all very
English country garden. Amidst all this reassuring comfort, it took me a while to realise that the door to the *en
suite* bathroom was, in fact, a prison gate with a dog collar and leash attached to its bars. On the walls in the
bathroom, there were photographs of hooded men
wearing stockings, and a Westward Bound calendar,
which for this month showed a woman riding a hooded
naked man.

Waiting for Sadi's return, I sipped a glass of sherry
(poured, no doubt, by Steve under Sadi's strict instruction), helped myself to some complimentary Hula
Hoops and browsed through their fetishwear catalogues;
we had been promised a ten per cent discount on anything we bought. The models included Sadi and Steve,
and the photos had been taken inside the house and in
their grounds. There were the traditional leather/rub-
ber basques, dresses and some more bizarre fetishwear.
The inflatable bra looked like a good idea. It definitely
knocked the Wonderbra into a hat. I wasn't quite sure
what I could do with a rubber nun's habit (unisex)
unless the Westward Bound Players were doing *Agnes of
God*. But I was absolutely certain about what I could do
with a pair of rubber briefs with internal solid penis.

There were a variety of hoods that catered for every
occasion bar christenings (but then, I suppose you drag

out the habit). There was an inflatable rubber hood with a tube for breathing which, I assumed, you'd blow up after you'd put it on. Or you could buy the Enclosure Helmet, which was made of thick rubber and had perspex eyes with a zipped and laced back.

They also sold wigs. Some like 'Bobby' and 'Marilyn' were modelled by transvestites. I was quite taken by the long-haired, blonde one called the 'Aphrodite', though it would have been more appropriately named the 'Bet Gilroy'. There were numerous bondage goods and many of them looked as if they should come with an Enhance warning. One item that certainly made an impression on me, was the shoe harness gag. This was a patent leather stiletto, attached by straps to the head and inserted in the mouth. Chic and unobtrusive, it seemed the perfect gift for a footwear fan like Ben.

Sadi returned.

'It's not really a bed and breakfast,' she said. 'If it was practical, we'd rather rent out the dungeon by the hour.' I got the feeling that Sadi felt that we should feel privileged for paying £175 to stay there. She insisted that she was not a hotelier and, therefore, we were to keep the place clean and tidy.

'I do not want to clean hairs out of the bath,' she said firmly.

I think she meant that she did not want to have to tell Steve to clean the hairs out of the bath.

Sadi led us down into the dungeon which was reached from the bedroom via a spiral staircase. At the top of the stairs, there was a sign which instructed the guests to 'Please leave the dungeon clean and tidy'. I didn't imagine that sign-writers got to use that template too often.

It took a while to adjust to the darkness of the dungeon. The carpet was black and the little light there was came from torchlike wall lights shining on to red-painted walls, casting a red glow around the room. The smell of leather was overwhelming. With obvious pride, Sadi went to each instrument of torture in turn and explained its workings with a sterling matter-of-factness.

On one wall hung enough weapons to make Miss Prim choke on her mortarboard. Alongside the usual paddles, tawses and whips (listen to me – 'usual'!) hung vicious-looking nipple clamps and weights, and, if they failed, a peg bag. There were wrist and ankle restraints, executioner's masks, inflatable rubber balls (I didn't ask) and bridles. Anything we used, instructed Sadi, was to be left out afterwards for Steve to clean. Straight after he'd got the pubes out of the bath.

These items were no more than a garnish to the serious hardware in the dungeon. Sadi showed us the rack, the gib and the electric chair.

'It feels like a Slendertone,' said Sadi, turning on the current.

Sadly, I knew that feeling.

There was a Maltese Cross with leather straps, a rotating spit, a bondage horse, various stocks and a school desk. Sadi proudly showed us their latest installation – ankle slings on a pulley. And to stretch my calf muscles, we could put a metal cage on my head and suspend it from the ceiling. Before she left, Sadi showed us the various keys for each of the locks.

As a security measure, we were to be locked into our room and dungeon. To get out, we had to ring a bell. This effectively put an end to the possibility of sneaking out for a quick fag. So, before we settled down in the dungeon we went off into town for something to eat with our forty cigarettes.

On our return, Steve showed us back in through the dungeon door and left. We soon had to call him back to retrieve one of their seventeen cats which had wedged itself under the rack. While trying to entice it out, he told us about a couple who had stayed there once who had a dog kennel with them. The husband forgot to shut the bedroom door and one of Sadi's tom cats had sprayed inside it. Incensed that the man had disobeyed her, the wife made him sleep in the kennel all night. Steve grabbed the cat and looked relieved. He wouldn't have to spend the night in the cat-litter tray.

There was a tape-deck in the dungeon. I put on some classical music while Dominic slipped into something more comfortable. For Dominic, 'something more comfortable' was a pink fluorescent wig and a pair of size nine stilettos. Were other people's honeymoons like this, I wondered, tying restraints to his ankles. These ankle cuffs were attached to either end of a two-foot pole which prevented him from closing his legs. The accumulative effect, as he staggered around the room, resembled a hormonally troubled Hermann Munster. It wasn't pleasant.

Dominic was itching to try the spit. The spit was a board which rotated horizontally through three hundred and sixty degrees, with the user secured by a series of leather straps. In the middle of the board, there was a hole cut out for the user's bum to be exposed after a half-turn.

'Lose the wig and I'll rotate,' I instructed.

Dominic did as he was told and lay on top of the spit. I strapped him on and turned the handle. Dominic rotated slowly. After a full circle I asked him how he felt.

'Like a kebab,' he answered, and I turned the handle another one hundred and eighty degrees and left him suspended face down while I read the framed Sacher-Masoch extracts on the wall.

Returning my attention to Dominic, I used a series of paddles and whips on his now vulnerable behind. I let him scream for a while and then turned him up the right way again.

'Did that turn you on?' I asked, though I could see full well that it hadn't.

'Mmm. So-so.'

Untying him from the spit, I led him to the electric chair and strapped him in. As I pulled the metal mask over his face, I asked him if he had a last request.

'A cigarette,' he said.

I pulled the handle.

'I can't feel anything,' he moaned from under the mask.

Then his wedding ring touched one of the metal studs conducting the current.

'It isn't very strong,' he complained.

'Are you turned on?'

'Well . . .'

I felt that I could have probably made the chair more exciting had I enacted a scenario. But I couldn't think of any to do with capital punishment. Ben was good at role-playing but I'm not sure if even he had one about an electric chair. I knew that he had a good one about the man from the electricity board. Something to do with Ben being caught fiddling the meter and then offering to pay with nature's own credit card.

Likewise, I was stuck for storylines when I tied Dominic to the Maltese Cross. He had been standing in the middle of the dungeon, naked save for a black hood over his head. He thought he looked menacingly sexy. I thought he looked like a match. Once fastened to the cross, there wasn't really a lot I could do with him on a Maltese theme. I tried pretending that the weights I had attached to his nipples were from Gozo but it didn't really add to the excitement.

I was worried that the problem may have been something to do with who was sub and who was dom. I mean, it's not really until you get into a dungeon that these things come into play. What if you both turn out to be sub? Who undoes the locks? More to the point, who does them up in the first place?

Every now and then, above the music (during the Maltese interlude it was the Hovis theme) we could hear Sadi and Steve wandering around the house. It felt strange that they knew that people were hiring out a room in their home to do questionable things to each other for sexual excitement. But then, they no doubt used it often themselves.

Dominic then went dom and tied me to the Bondage Horse. This was like a massage table with a raised section close to one end. Firmly trussed, I lay on my front with my stomach over the raised section, thus pushing my not unsubstantial bum out even further. The joy of the Bondage Horse was that, once I was bound up, I didn't have to do anything. Not that I do much anyway. But it was nice to have an excuse.

After a while I lost all sensation in my tethered limbs, so Dominic untied me. Continuing this theme of restraint without strain, I tried the ankle pulleys. As my legs were hoisted into the air, I felt a strange sense of *déjà vu*. Pushing the feeling to one side, I permitted Dominic to have his evil dom way with me.

Suddenly, I knew what the feeling was. Back in the seventies, my mother had bought a very similar device from Ronco under the guise of it being a slimming aid. Daily, around lunchtime, my mother would slip into her leotard, hang the pulley over the living-room door-handle and attach it to her wrists and ankles. In this position she could quite happily exercise while watching 'Paint Along with Nancy Kominsky'. In time, the door-handle worked away from its moorings. One day, during a tricky sweep with a purple tone, it fell off completely and Mrs Shirley Churchill surprised herself. It's funny how your mind wanders during sex because the next thing I knew I was having an orgasm to the climax of the '1812 Overture'.

At one time the idea of hiring a dungeon for a bit of light SM and bondage would have been extremely exciting. But my afternoon with the Moonglow Dining Club had pretty much killed off the eroticism around it and the whole experience felt quite contrived. Being tied to your bedpost by your partner is one thing but paying to use a rotating spit in somebody else's home where many have rotated before is another. It made me feel slightly queasy.

Afterwards, I was desperate for a post-coital cigarette. Untied from the pulley, I went off and committed the most masochistic act of the day. I stood under a cold shower and smoked, hoping that the running water would somehow prevent the smell from reaching the dominant nostrils of Mistress Sadi.

Chapter 20

TINKERBELLED

Fed up with people hitting each other, I made my second attempt at spiritually unblocking my sexual U-bend. This time it involved Joachim, a German sexologist in Bristol who promised to bring enlightenment on the secrets of ancient and modern sexuality. On the phone, Joachim told me that sexuality is the most creative and empowering force available to us. Joachim's therapy incorporated sexual secrets from Tibetan, Indian and Chinese Taoist philosophies. I was going to be released from all my inhibitions by relaxing, with a number of other people, in a hot tub.

Ben read his leaflet and wasn't convinced. 'How many time-proven Tibetan sexual secrets do you think you're going to learn in a hot tub?' he asked. I despaired about his lack of spiritual depth and told him so.

'I am spiritual,' he protested.

'Why, because you know all the words to that song by

the Singing Nun? Look, it says here that for only £100 he can help you create an orgasm in every cell of your body and show you how to attract and keep the right man,' I said, a little irritated.

'I'll tell you for free. Buy yourself a mains vibrator and never wear patchouli.'

Early on a Sunday morning, I found myself puffing up and down the hills of Clifton on my way to Joachim's home. Pausing to ring the sweat from my aura, I spotted a couple of free love-ers obviously heading in the same direction as myself, and Ben's words rang in my head. Never wear patchouli. The spell was broken and my cynicism came flooding back. Dominique a-knicker knicker, I sang to myself as I walked up the hill. But I couldn't remember how it went after that . . .

Joachim greeted me at the door and took me up to his top-floor flat. He asked me to take off my shoes before entering his pale pink living-room. Inside, John and Sarah, the hippy couple, had already shucked their Birkenstocks and were sitting on the couch next to Steve, a muscle man with a whiff of bouncer about him. Next to him was Carol, a Joachim-junkie and, occupying my favoured 'huddled in the corner, twitching' spot, was Peter.

Joachim asked each of us in turn what we expected to gain from the day. Carol started crying before my bum had even hit a bean bag. Between sobs, she admitted that her parents had been bastards and now she felt emotionally withdrawn. Handing her a handkerchief, I felt she could do with withdrawing a bit more; but, before I could say anything, Peter burst into tears too. He was angry he said, really, really angry at how inconsiderate people were towards him. He wanted to learn how to express his anger. He seemed oblivious to the fact that he'd shouted all this.

Sarah wanted to learn to direct her sexual energy towards a creative end. To me that could only mean one thing – body painting – but, predictably, Joachim was impressed. Her partner, John, wanted creativity too and a better sex life, while Steve just seemed to be under the influence of steroid abuse.

I felt all eyes turn on me.

'I'd just like to want sex more.'

There was silence. They wanted more from me.

'I'm just as happy to read a book.'

Still nothing.

What did these people want me to say? That I had an overwhelming desire to knot myself a macramé yoni?

'I'd like to be more active.'

Joachim decided that I had a lot of angry emotions towards my partner.

'No, I'm just lazy.'

We were told that the exercises we were going to learn before going to the hot tub would help us unchain our sexual energy. First, we all had to stand in a circle and vigorously shake our hands with our knees bent. Then we had to shake our heads and shoulders as well. After five minutes of this, we were told to place our hands about five inches apart and feel the energy. Now, it's true you can feel a power surge but, cynic as ever, I remembered at school, pushing my hand against a wall for a while and then watching as my arm involuntarily rose in the air. I felt this might be working under the same principle.

While we were feeling the power, Joachim asked us to clench our sphincter muscles.

'Feel the power surge!' he enthused. 'Squeeze your vaginas! Flip your penises!'

Suddenly aware that I was in a room full of men flipping their penises, I lost concentration and the power slipped away. The next exercise had us walking around the room in a circle like a Pentonville exercise period. We had to massage the neck of the person in front of us. As the person in front of me was at least a foot taller, I settled for making a stab at his shoulder blades.

Then we had to dance. I don't know why five minutes of doing The Monkey to a SingalongaRavi album should elevate you to a higher plain but, invariably on the path to realness, the moment comes when you have to frug. This time we did it in pairs, one half frantically aping the movements of the other. As I danced, a blinding revelation hit me. Punk had happened. I knew now that my Jefferson Airplane albums would never leave the attic again.

We finished dancing. Flushed from my spiritual insight, I listened as Joachim filled us in on the basics of their philosophy. Joachim told us that Christianity had split the mind and body and made people feel guilty about sex. He said that sex was innocent and that his programme was designed to make us feel the same way. I thought about all the things I had been doing in recent months and felt that the Christians might have a point.

We then had to meditate to get our Love Circuit flowing. To help us along, Joachim brought out a circuit diagram showing a couple making love. With our Third Eye, we had to imagine a golden ball making its way through our alimentary system, stopping off at the heart and genitals along the way. Although I did feel a burning sensation, it jumped my genitals completely and my Love Plug blew a fuse before the circuit was through. John was experiencing the same problem. Joachim explained that the exercise was to help us focus our minds the way we should do when we make love.

'People,' he said, 'have a terrible habit of thinking about everything else but the actual act. Like going shopping in Sainsbury's.'

Milk, bread, Brasso, I thought and suddenly remembered we should be meditating. Joachim walked around the room, lightly touching people's foreheads. When he came to John, John claimed that he felt like he was being pushed back. Sarah jumped in and informed us that John was a forceps delivery.

'Ah, yes,' said Joachim. 'You are reliving a birth memory. It is good.'

'I had a similar experience the last time I was rebirthed,' said John, delighted. Why was I not the tiniest bit surprised that John had been rebirthed?

Accepting that my Love Circuit was a crystal set compared to John and Sarah's Apple Macs, I went off for a cigarette. Naturally, when I returned, Joachim told me that smokers have a very low aura.

'It's amazing,' said Joachim, 'The radioactive material in cigarettes is so powerful that even if you don't smoke, standing next to a smoker or even a packet of cigarettes can affect your aura.'

Everyone looked at me like I was a murderer. Even just the packet? Had none of these people ever been into a newsagents?

Steve admitted that during the last exercise he hadn't felt anything, anywhere. I had noticed that he was having trouble digesting Joachim's belief that seminal emission saps a man's strength. (According to Joachim, when a man comes, his body is fooled into thinking that it is making babies, thereby taking away the body's nutrients.) Steve looked the type to have let the odd teaspoon's worth fall on barren ground.

'Do other drugs have the same effect as cigarettes?' he asked.

'If you mean marijuana,' said Joachim, 'then yes.'

Steve looked a bit sheepish. He'd clearly been taking a few short cuts to spiritual enlightenment.

With an aura that resembled a pair of fishnet tights, I struggled on through the next few exercises. We had to picture our genitals and think about what we felt about them. 'If you don't like them,' said Joachim, 'throw them into the universe. You can have new ones.'

I pictured my vagina floating through space to the sound of 'The Blue Danube' and thought better of it. Everybody else kept their parts on the launching pad too, although John confessed to feeling angry about his penis. He had been forcibly circumcised at nine.

Joachim was triumphant. 'Excellent. Excellent. I knew this to be the problem and do you know why?'

No-one did.

'It was obvious when you jumped over your genitals in the meditation.'

What about my jump? I'd never been angry with my vulva. But maybe it was angry with me. We'd have to talk later.

In the meantime, Joachim asked us to visualise our genitals as a colour. In a triumphant moment of inspiration, I came up with pink. Most of the others favoured saffron and while I pondered on the reason why, Joachim decided we were now ready to choose our partners for the hot tub. But first we had to discuss any feelings we may have about it.

Peter and Carol, who had been quiet in the other exercises, now came into their own. Carol having been to twenty of these hot tubs said she was very worried that the men in the group might start thrashing around in their anger and that she had felt intimidated by this in the past. I started to wonder what I had got myself into. By comparison, I felt the swingers and the fetishists were easy numbers. These people were weird.

However, Joachim was pleased that she had brought this matter up and said that although people should express their feelings, they should be respectful of how others would feel. Peter took this as his cue to share his worries.

'I'd like to work with a woman in the tub,' he said, 'but I'm worried about sexual assault.'

Carol, having stopped her sobbing for a couple of minutes, was confused. 'What do you mean?'

Peter elucidated. 'I'm worried I might rape her.'

Get some therapy, I wanted to scream but waited for Joachim's spiritual response. He seemed slightly put off his stroke and just assured Peter that he wouldn't let this happen. We then had to spin around and around, stop and choose our partner by looking them in the eye. If they looked back at you, they were the right people. Guess who was staring at me? Peter, who appeared to have jump leads attached to his Love Circuit. I fixed my gaze on Steve. Thankfully, he looked back. Carol ended up with Peter and started crying again.

The tub was a couple of miles away in a quiet bunga-low. As you entered the womb-like room, the smell of incense was overwhelming, there were many lit candles and it was incredibly warm. There was a tape crackling in the background and just as I was about to tell Joachim there was something wrong with it, Carol asked me if I liked the heartbeat music.

Joachim sent us off to change. I still wasn't sure how the tub was meant to work or what it was really for. From what I could gather, the idea was to sit in the tub, hyperventilate to the point of nausea and then experience much relief when the dizziness stopped. I soon caught on though, when I came out of the changing room and found myself to be the only person with a swimming costume on.

'Why are you wearing that?' asked Joachim.

'Because I wouldn't feel comfortable naked,' came my obvious reply.

'This is all about rebirthing and no-one's ever been born in a swimming costume.'

I wanted to tell him that, according to Ben, Esther Williams was, but Carol had stopped crying for a minute and I didn't want to break the spell.

I kept my costume on.

We then all climbed into the tub. It was boiling and soon my skin had an attractive mauvish tone to it. Taking it in turns to lie back in our partner's arms, we did some heavy breathing which wasn't easy for a forty-a-day Marlboro smoker like myself. I wheezed through the exercise. The others all seemed real pros. Sarah and John looked like they had been born to rebirth. Using snorkels, they submerged themselves completely. Carol was off again, her sobbing building to a crescendo. I couldn't work out if it was because she had been rebirthed twenty-one times or because she had forgotten her snorkel.

I did feel light-headed and tingly all over but again, nothing was happening with my Love Circuit, I still didn't know the secret of how to have an orgasm in every cell of my body and I didn't feel reborn. About an hour later, when my whole body was wrinkled, we stopped and all shared our feelings. It became obvious that everyone, apart from Steve and I, felt wonderful. I felt nothing. I'm sure Ben got more from sitting in the hot tub with Darryl's toe up his arse at the tower party.

I left disappointed but determined not to be defeated. I would give spiritual sex one more chance. My final attempt at reaching Nirvana saw me on a dull afternoon in Kilburn having my perineum stimulated by a complete stranger. Actually, before it happened, I didn't even know that it was my perineum. It was the same with Liechtenstein. I knew it existed, I'd just never felt the need to go and look it up on a map.

I had booked myself an appointment with The Kaizen Sexual Training Programme. Initially, Ben had been quite keen to come with me but when he found out that Patrick, who runs the programme, was a Taoist, he changed his mind. As Joachim had pointed out to Steve, Taoists believe that ejaculation causes the depletion of the male fire energy or yang. Therefore, a man of thirty should be aiming to ejaculate only once every ten to twelve couplings. Ben thought that was okay as he'd faked an orgasm in the past. But masturbation was completely out on the same grounds and Ben adamantly refused to cut back on what he called his 'quality time'. He'd never make it as a Taoist anyway. Aside from having a yang drought at UN intervention levels, his knowledge of yin extended only as far as his Judy

Garland cut-out doll book. (I must just say, helping him to cut out all those Seconals was a chore.)

I went to Kilburn with some trepidation: I couldn't face any more heavy breathing or fused Love Circuits. I was convinced that I would chat politely about techniques and maybe ask for the finer points to be explained to me with the aid of anatomically correct dolls.

My meeting with Patrick began with a discussion on the state of my sexual relationship. Although the past few months had seen me in a variety of very odd sexual situations, I did think that, in my relationship with Dominic, things were going slightly off the boil. It's a problem I have when I feel secure in a relationship: I start not to bother. For me, domestic bliss means clean sex and a dirty housecoat. Aside from that, my activities over the last few months had taken their toll. People use sex to take their mind off the stresses of work. How was I meant to take my mind off what I was doing?

It wasn't just me. Dominic wasn't above reproach either. I was beginning to feel that he saw me as a milking machine with eyeliner – quick, cold and never a drop spilled. Patrick nodded sagely as I poured my heart out and there was no stopping me. I said that Dominic had a problem in coming too quickly. I didn't think his ejaculation was exactly premature, just a little bit previous. Patrick felt that I had to take some of the blame for what was going wrong in my bedroom.

'Your orgasms are your own responsibility,' he said. 'Nobody else's.'

I bridled at the inference that I wasn't doing my bit. I arched my back sometimes.

Patrick then offered me a practical demonstration of his Taoist practices. I accepted, trying to think of him as just a sexual Avon Lady. He explained the procedure. First he would give me a Taoist massage and then stop and ask me if I wanted to go further. Going further meant stimulating my sexual energies starting with my perineum. As I've said, I had to ask of its whereabouts hoping against hope that it would be situated below the knee. Patrick told me where it was. It suddenly occurred to me that bestiality shouldn't necessarily be struck off my sexual exploration list. Ben could start doing the fieldwork immediately.

Patrick asked me to take off my clothes.

'All of them?' I squeaked.

He pointed out that it would be pretty impractical not to. As a woman who has been known to keep her tights on during intercourse, I couldn't see how. He explained that the massage oil would go everywhere. I calmed myself down. Just like being at my gynaecologist's, I thought. But then *he* lets me keep my bra on and doesn't burn incense.

The massage lasted about half an hour and I needed every second to try and prise my knees apart. It was quite pleasant, but any time Patrick's hands went below my navel rigor mortis set in. Patrick then asked me if I was ready to go on to the next stage which is where we came in with my newly found perineum under the spotlight. Well, while you're down there, I thought, you might as well. As he massaged old Peri, I was told to repeatedly clench my vaginal and anal muscles. That was easy, unclenching them was the difficult bit. I also had to breathe deeply. I suddenly realised I hadn't breathed at all in the previous thirty minutes. Trying to co-ordinate clenches and breaths was a bit like trying to pat your head and rub your belly at the same time.

He then moved on to the sexual energy centre situated just below and around the clitoris. I think I must have been hyperventilating at that point because I can't remember if my perineum had been abandoned or not. I generally find it difficult to have an orgasm and, despite Patrick's expertise, I was sure his wrist would go before I came. And yet in a matter of minutes – pow! Pot Noodles have taken longer to stir. Let me draw you a picture. When Disney Time comes on there's fireworks over the castle, a fairy flies out and pixie dust streams off her wand. It was like that. I'd been Tinkerbelled.

Ben asked afterwards, 'Didn't you just feel like you'd been to a middle-class prostitute?' (The session costs £60.)

'He was a professional,' I replied, none too sure that I hadn't. 'Anyway my bigger concern is telling Dominic.'

Like me, Dominic had also believed that it was going to be a strictly hands-off affair.

Ben offered some words of comfort. 'As you said, the man's a professional. It's the same as when your car goes. You don't mind Dominic having a quick shufty under the bonnet, but occasionally you have to take it into Kwik-Fit for a proper service.'

With that, Ben was off, singing 'Dominique, a-knicker, knicker' as he went.

Chapter 21

FWOWING UP

Baby Girl Ben sat in the high-chair and Mummy Hazel High-Heels fed her her din-dins. As Mummy knew that Baby Girl Ben wasn't really a baby, she forewent the Cow & Gate Braised Beef and Carrots and gave her ice cream and pineapple instead. This made Baby Girl Ben happy, although not happy enough to pick up her rattle and shake it. Mummy had said that the rattle got on her nerves and was strictly forbidden anywhere other than the nursery. Baby Girl Ben took this as a warning. There was a sign on a shelf in the nursery which said, 'Rule No. 1: Mummy is always right. Rule No. 2: Refer to Rule No. 1.' Stuck in the high-chair, Baby Girl Ben was in no position to argue.

Ben hadn't always been so reticent.

'No, not under any circumstances. No, no, no!' he said, with a finality that I thought I could break in seconds.

'For the sake of journalistic veracity, you have to,' I argued.

'I'm sorry, I'm not wetting myself.'

And on that point, surprisingly enough, he was not to be moved. Nevertheless, I had scored something of a victory. Ben had agreed to go to the Hush-A-Bye-Baby Club and experience the view from the other side of the cot bars.

From the start of my journey through the sexual underbelly of England, the subject of adult babyhood had sat in the background like a filled nappy. The smell wouldn't go away and somebody would have to attend to it. When we had first run into the babies in their crèche at the Safer Planet Sex Ball, Ben had defended them, probably in the belief that he would never have to sit in the high-chair himself. I never believed that he missed the train to the Muir Reform Academy accidentally and, as an act of revenge, I had secretly sent away in his name for more details on the sexual infantilism scene.

The letter which arrived from the Hush-A-Bye-Baby Club was headed 'Dear Baby'. It explained that the club had been running for five years and had around 200 members across the world, mostly male. The facilities available at the nurseries were extensive. In the first nursery there was a large white wooden cot, an extra large pink high-chair, a pushchair, a rocking horse, storybooks, videos, nappy pail, changing mat, baby oil and baby powder. In the second nursery, also known as the cradle room, there was a rocking cradle, a play pen, another highchair and things that were available 'in more traditional nurseries'. Not including, of course, traditional babies.

When Mummy Hazel listed some of the clothing

available at the club, I wondered what kind of traditional nurseries she'd been in. Alongside the bibs, bonnets, mittens and bootees there was a rubber bondage bag with sleeves on the inside, lots of leather straps, ropes, handcuffs, padlocks and a straitjacket. Maybe the nursery was situated in a difficult catchment area.

Mummy was specific about what services she did and didn't offer. 'While you may expect me to feed you in the high-chair or give you a bottle or a spanking, or ensure that you are securely strapped in, you may not expect any sexual service from me.' Of course not, that would be weird. She said that, because the nurseries were situated in her home, adult babies were expected to be well protected and not wet the furniture. Wetting oneself was allowed but 'soiling' was strictly forbidden. 'I don't change wet nappies or administer enemas.'

Mummy also offered a full mail-order service for those unfortunate families, normally on welfare, who could not afford to send their offspring to a nursery. For parents who fretted that their at-home children would be missing out on the educational leg-up that nurseries offer, Mummy had provided a full range of Snuggledown Stories which trashed the low aspirations of penny dreadfuls like *Spot the Dog*. There were hundreds of Snuggledown Stories to choose from including *It's An Ill Wind* by Rose, *The Damp Patch* by Paul, and a whole host of titles from the prolific pen of Prissy such as *Let Me Dwess Oo Up*, *My Baby Daddy* and *It's MY Teddy*.

(It's a little known fact that, in the late thirties, Metro-Goldwyn-Mayer tried to option Prissy's magnum opus *Hotel Baby World* in the hope of filming it as a big-budget musical fantasy which would utilise the then-new Technicolor process. Fearing that the studio would vulgarise her work, Prissy turned them down and MGM were forced to go with the vastly inferior *Wizard of Oz*.)

The oh-too-common occurrence of adult babies being caught shoplifing in Mothercare could become a thing of the past if they would only choose to mail-order from Mummy. From polycotton pixie party dresses to satin yoke-bonnets, they were all there. Items were priced to suit all pockets from fifty pence for an extra large nappy pin to just under £1,000 for a wooden cot with bars. I could even send off £25 for a hypnotherapy tape that would help Ben get over his block about wetting himself.

I phoned Mummy Hazel to book Ben into the nursery although I was rather worried by the fact that nowhere on her information sheet did she actually state that she was a registered child-minder. My fears were not allayed by Mummy Hazel having to ask me whether Ben was a baby boy or a baby girl. Of course he was a baby boy. I hoped she wouldn't still be confused when she met him and make him wear one of those nappies with the extra padding in the wrong place.

I thought about booking Ben in for a five-day holiday stay at the nursery which cost £400. Although that seemed expensive, I reasoned with myself that I would save some money by being able to buy cigarettes with his DSS milk tokens. Still uncertain about the actual depths of Mummy's maternalism, I settled for an initial two-hour visit which cost £20 an hour plus £20 for clothes hire. I opted for clothes hire as I didn't want Ben to get anything down his 0–12 dungarees.

The day that he went, I felt the wrench that all working mothers must feel when forced to hand over their offspring to professional carers. If only I'd had a body-harness bed restraint in my office, he wouldn't have had to go. I could hardly work that day for thinking about him. That and the fact that I spent the afternoon sitting in a pub garden. I know I could have made him a matinée jacket while I was sitting there but I was too cross-eyed to crochet. I couldn't help it. It's the Medea in me.

When he came home later, white of face and milky of breath, I knew he was upset because he toyed with his Alphabetti Spaghetti and scribbled over the face of the Fat Controller. Finally, when he tried to stab me with one of his Play People, I knew we had to talk about what had happened. Clutched to my bosom, he told his story, taking deep breaths to fight back the tears. His account was slightly garbled, after all, it was a big day for the little boy. So I have done my best to reconstruct the day's events as they were told to me. This, then, is Baby Ben's story.

When Ben awoke on his first morning of nursery, the first thing he did was throw up, or as paediatric experts such as Prissy would term it 'fwow up'. This was not, as one may think, due to an inexpertly mixed bottle of SMA formula. It was because Ben had finally realised the perverseness of what he was about to do and was struck with terror. The sensible option after such an experience would have been to drink lots of fluids, but Ben was determined that his bladder would remain in a Saharan state until the whole ordeal was over. Under no circumstances would he allow himself to be caught short in a Peaudouce 2–3 years trainer-nappy.

The nursery was situated in Kent, site of so many of our sexual escapades and, incidentally, home to Ben's mother's eight-berth caravan. He took the train there and, as the Ramsgate Express flew through the Garden of England,˙ he pondered how he had let himself be baby-talked into spending the afternoon wearing incontinence pads when he could have been playing swing-ball with the Family Ben outside their holiday home on Plot C11.

On arriving at his destination, he had been told to phone Mummy Hazel and await further instructions. Having arrived half an hour early, he went to McDonald's and toyed with the idea of ordering a Happy Meal to get himself into the mood. There was a children's party going on in the burger bar and Ben watched queasily as the staff brought out a couple of high-chairs for the younger party-goers. Such a foreshadowing of the events to come proved too unsettling and Ben walked the streets until the appointed hour.

He phoned Mummy Hazel and she arranged to pick him up in front of the station. When she arrived, he told her he would have been happy to have got a cab.

'We don't give out our address for security reasons,' she said.

This was odd, as her front door had appeared on television just a few days earlier, during a profile of the group's activities. In fact, Mummy Hazel courted media interest and had, a few weeks earlier, been the subject of an in-depth piece in the *Independent*. She felt that the more the subject of sexual infantilism in adults was discussed, then the less taboo it would become. Soon may that day come, but I don't think when it does I will feel all that comfortable pushing a trolley round Safeways with a twelve-stone thirty-year-old sitting in the child seat with a teething ring. I've had a thought: after enlightenment, will adult babies go for half on the bus?

Mummy Hazel didn't look particularly maternal to Ben. He assumed that she would be an ample breasted, apple-cheeked earth mother in a smock. Instead, she looked like a small, dark, middle-aged heavy metal fan.

Although unprompted, Ben felt the need to explain some of his sexual credentials. He briefly detailed the sexual odyssey in which he had taken part and mentioned my visit to Miss Prim. It turned out that, only the previous week, Mummy Hazel had been to a barbecue held by the headmistress.

'She's got big wrists,' said Mummy Hazel of the venerable pedagogue. 'But Miss Prim said she'd never seen a spanking technique as good as mine and spent the whole evening trying to learn it.'

Ben couldn't remember whether spanking was part of the package, or an optional extra and asked, 'What can I expect from this afternoon?'

'To be treated like a baby,' said Mummy Hazel simply.

Arriving at her house, she warned Ben about her dogs. She claimed that their barks were worse than their bites, but when she opened the door and two big snarling monsters leapt out, Ben was convinced that the headline in the following day's Kent Gleaner would read, 'Adult Baby Mauled In Pram'. Ben had expected the house to be detached due to the covert activities of its inhabitants but it was slap bang in the middle of a terrace.

Mummy Hazel invited Ben into her kitchen, where a middle-aged woman was parcelling up rubber knickers for mail-order clients. The woman, named Margaret, had been the nurse in charge of the crèche at the Ball. A big dummy sat on the table portentously and Ben relented on his no-liquid rule by allowing Mummy Hazel to make him a cup of coffee to stave off the moment when he would actually have to go into the nursery.

His heart sank when Mummy Hazel informed him that she didn't start counting the two hours of the appointment until the client was inside the nursery walls and he downed his coffee quickly. He had begun to realise that Mummy Hazel was committed to providing a good service. She asked him if he'd ever phoned a credit card sex line as she was thinking of starting one. He said no, which was a lie. (It truly is a pathetic sight to watch a man phone up a dirty chatline and try and charge it to his BHS Storecard.) Mummy Hazel was concerned by the way that other chatlines ripped off their customers by making them listen to, and charging them for, minutes of nonessential information before coming up with the goods.

Finishing his coffee, Ben was led upstairs into the nursery. This was nursery one, as described in the letter, though the rocking horse was sadly absent. The walls were covered in fluffy bear-type wallpaper and there was a whole host of fluffy bear-type animals on the floor and on the mansize cot in the corner. Above the fireplace, there was a delicate painting of a woman holding a leash attached to the exposed erection of an adult baby transvestite. This painting made Ben feel glad that he was going to be an adult baby boy. Transvestism just seemed so odd on top of all that.

'So are you going to be a boy or a girl?' asked Mummy Hazel. 'Or are you going to let me choose?'

'A boy,' said Ben firmly. And then, 'Oh, you choose.'

'I think you're a baby girl,' said Mummy Hazel, which was fortunate as she had a baby girl's outfit hanging on the back of the door.

She rummaged through a chest of drawers by the side
of the cot looking for pink bootees to go with the outfit.
Ben was then told to take off all his clothes. When he
was nude, she laid out an incontinence pad on the cot
and told him to lie on it. As he did so, she turned on a
musical chime hanging above the cot and quickly sprin-
kled baby powder over his manhood (babyhood?). She
fastened the nappy then looked around for the right
size PVC pull-ons. She held up an array of rubber knickers and Ben chose the largest size which were still a tight
fit around the thigh, which, I suppose, is the point. Just
before putting them on him, Mummy Hazel took a
sticker off them. On it was written a man's name.

'He never bothered to collect them,' she said.

Ben cringed at the thought of wearing another man's
pull-ons and tried to distract himself with the musical
chimes.

The outfit itself was a triumph in pink broderie
Anglaise. The top was a baby doll extending just past
Ben's navel to the tops of the matching pink broderie
anglaise knickers. To top it off, she tied a white cotton
bonnet around his spinning head and let him look at
the results in the mirror on the wall at the foot of the
cot.

'There,' said Mummy Hazel, 'isn't that better now
you've got rid of all your nasty adult clothes?'

Ben looked at himself and thought the effect would
have been better if he'd also got rid of his nasty adult
two-day beard growth. 'I can't wet myself,' he said, by
way of something to say.

'It isn't compulsory,' said Mummy Hazel, 'but if you
do the other thing, it's an on-the-spot £200 fine.'

Ben clenched his sphincter stoically and Hazel left

him to watch the documentary which featured her front door. In it, one of her regular clients explained how he came to the club to get rid of stress. Being an adult baby, he said (wearing a blonde wig), makes it a lot easier to go into work and sack people. As always with this type of documentary, he said that a lot of his friends didn't know about his activities. Would it be stating the obvious to say that they do now? Surely these people can't think that *all* of their friends are watching the other channel?

Mummy Hazel returned with a list of videos that Ben could watch from the cot. Most of them were along the TV torment lines of *Punished in Panties*, but there were a few of a slightly different nature.

'Is there anything you'd like to see?' asked Mummy Hazel.

'There is actually,' said Ben.

Mummy Hazel brightened. Maybe Ben was warming to being a baby girl. She didn't know quite how much. 'Which one?'

'Walt Disney's *Beauty and the Beast.*'

Going off to look for it, she asked Ben if he wanted a big dummy or a regular dummy. Feeling that there wasn't enough room in the cot for two big dummies, he plumped for regular. Before going to the nursery, Ben had confessed to me that he had a morbid fear of having a dummy in his mouth, but when it arrived he took to it like a rubber duck to water sports. With the dummy in his mouth, he didn't have to do baby-talk which was his other big worry beforehand. Dominic had tried coaching him with a few 'coochie-coos'; Ben had run out of the room screaming. Likewise, he wasn't too happy when we presented him with a christening spoon the day before going.

Aside from being a keen Disney fan, Ben had another reason for picking *Beauty and the Beast*. He was very keen to remove any sexual content from the afternoon. He had noticed a large selection of magazines on the shelf above the television. Getting up to see if they had a back issue of *Twinkle*, he found that they were all porn magazines. It dawned on him that Mummy Hazel was leaving him alone with a video so that he could play with himself. He wasn't prepared to do that. Anyway, he couldn't get the press studs undone on his nappy.

Mummy Hazel brought the film back and then promised to come in halfway through and feed him. As he watched the credits roll up, he had the realisation that he was just like Brer Rabbit in the briar patch. Although I had arranged this whole thing as a punishment for him, he found that there was actually nothing more comfortable than laying in a cot watching cartoons and being fed. He was born into a briar patch just like it.

Mummy Hazel came in to feed him at half-time. She knew she was on to a losing battle trying to convince him he was a baby girl and she quickly dropped the diddums bit and just shovelled in the ice cream as he sat in the pink high-chair singing along to 'Be My Guest'. He also had a trainer mug with a picture of Winnie the Pooh on the side, although she didn't insist that he drink from it in front of her. When she left, he found out that it was nice to be able to watch TV lying down and still drink at the same time.

When the film finished, Mummy Hazel said that Ben could go and sit in the pram in the garden. As this was only a terraced house, to do so would be to invite the hostile attention of the neighbours. Ben was game. He had managed to lose his bootees, so Mummy Hazel skirted around for a pair of shoes. She came up with a choice of two. One was a simple pair of men's sandals and the other, a pair of very nice, according to Ben, black patent women's shoes, low at the front with a court heel and a bow which tied around the ankles. Knowing Ben's predilection, do I have to say which pair he went for?

The shoes were new and Ben had to navigate the stairs carefully as the soles were slipping on the carpet. He was shocked to hear a man's voice coming from the kitchen and thought, what if he sees me like this, then realised that chances were the man would probably be wearing the same shoes himself later on.

Indeed, as Ben passed him by on the way to the garden, the man murmured, 'Nice shoes'.

Mummy Hazel said that on this occasion she wouldn't strap Ben in, in case he panicked. He sat in the garden for about ten minutes, daring the neighbours to peek through their Venetians. Finally, it occurred to him that he was getting nothing from the whole experience aside from having the blood supply to his legs cut off because of the pull-ons.

He went back inside where Mummy Hazel offered to feed him a bottle which he declined.

'You're not really into this dependency thing,' said Mummy Hazel.

Ben confessed that he wasn't and went upstairs to change, hearing Mummy Hazel behind him, telling the shoe-admirer that, yes, of course, he could go in the pram.

Ben came down in his adult clothes and Mummy Hazel offered him a cup of tea and a lift to the station. She apologised for not taking him into the cradle room.

'Margaret has been cleaning it up,' she explained. 'The baby who was using it always makes such a mess.'

Ben blanched.

'It's just baby powder,' she reassured him. 'He gets it everywhere.'

Driving back to the station, she told Ben that BT had closed down her 0898 phone lines, which was why she was intending to start up a private credit card line. She had been making around £1,000 a week from them.

'I've got a good mind to send them my CV,' said Mummy Hazel. 'I'm a doctor.'

She explained how, in the eighties, she had had enough of working long hours as a biochemist on a poorly paid research grant. Her boyfriend at the time, who was a transvestite, said that as she was handy with a Singer, she should make clothes for drag queens. She put out an advert and found that one of the items most requested was a baby doll just like the one Ben had been wearing. She had taken a business course and knew that you should never turn down the chance to be the first into a new market. She diversified into the adult baby line and the rest is history.

Admiring her entrepreneurial spirit, Ben came back to London disappointed about the phone lines. He'd wanted to rush home and listen to 0898 *Dominated! Humiliated! Cissyfied!* and relive the day again. I think that's why he was so vicious with the Play People.

ALL SHAGGED OUT

'Have you thought about *Overground*?' asked Ben, draining the bottle.

'What is it?' I asked, similarly finishing my beer and adding the bottle to the vast collection before me on the table.

'It's a contact magazine for amputee seekers.'

'Do I have to have a leg off?'

'Think of the weight you'd lose,' said Ben, waving at the waiter to attract his attention.

Ben didn't need to wave really to attract anyone's attention as we were sitting in a rather trendy bar in Islington and he was wearing my bra. Once again my bosoms had gone all Pavlovian on me and I'd taken off my brassière in public to offset the feelings of ennui. Not to be outdone, Ben had picked up my discarded Gypsy and was wearing it over his jacket.

'We're getting a bit silly, aren't we?' said Ben. We looked at each other and started to laugh.

The casual onlooker would have guessed that Ben's remark about being silly referred to our state of (un)dress, but it was more than that. The whole of our lives were becoming ridiculous. It was time to call it a day.

The reason Ben brought up the amputee club was because, at the last minute, the SM gymkhana was cancelled. But I didn't write off to *Overground* and I didn't go along with the Polaireian Society to visit underwear factories with other corsetry fetishists. Nor did I join the Acorn Society (for fans of the glans of the penis) or the International Mackintosh Society (for raincoat enthusiasts). And feeling that Dominic had met the TV remit in Miss Sadi's dungeon, and that Ben had kind of crossdressed in the bar, I didn't subject either of them to a transvestite make-over. And speaking of transvestites, if I accidentally bumped into my friend Saucy Mark in the street, I'd have to tell him that, no, I was no longer looking for action. It was time to call a halt to my odyssey. I was shagged out.

Ben, too, was reluctant to go on. Spending half a year pretending to be heterosexual had taken its toll. He claimed that he no longer sat with his legs crossed, had taken to belching and couldn't remember the tune to 'The Ladies Who Lunch'. He told me that if I wanted him to continue faking heterosexuality, I'd have to start faking homosexuality, which in this instance meant having my head shaved and spending the night on Hampstead Heath. The idea held some appeal but I didn't think as a heterosexual it was my place to comment on the sex lives of gay men or lesbians. Anyway, gay men and lesbians are too often defined by what they do in their bedrooms (or on the Heath). And besides, I didn't know the tune to 'The Ladies Who Lunch' in the first place.

However, some of the people I met along the way were reluctant to let me go without a fight. Joachim, the hot-tub guru, wouldn't take no for an answer. He rang me several times and whatever tack I took with him – angry, hysterical, withdrawn – he just interpreted it as proof that I was in further need of his hot tub. No doubt Carol was still sitting in there, on to rebirth number thirty, looking like a prune and blowing her nose.

The Ring of Confidentes were even more persistent callers. To get rid of Pete on one occasion, I told him that Ben had left me. There was a respectful day's wait before his partner, Dave, phoned me to see if I was ready to climb into the saddle again. 'Too soon,' I said, letting him down gently. But I knew he'd be back. I know swingers work to a different timetable, but even Party Susan's Adam was allowed six weeks to mourn for Moira. Erotic Eats wanted me back for seconds, Gillian The Punctuator still knocked out a note now and then, and I was fast running out of space in my album for my collection of pudendas on Polaroid.

A magazine also offered to give me my own column on sex. You'll understand that I wasn't too thrilled about it when I tell you that it was Auntie Claire's column in *Footsy*. A while after I'd moaned about not receiving any replies from prospective foot worshippers, pedi-paeans began arriving on my doormat by the sackload. There was also a letter from head honcho Dennis offering me gainful employment stepping into Auntie Claire's shoes. I tried putting my foot in a cauliflower cheese and binned all correspondence. It was all over.

Be careful of what you wish for – it may come true. There's truth in that cliché. As I've said before, some of the things I've done in the line of research involved living out some of my sexual fantasies. And yet, in over six months, I amassed a grand total of two orgasms directly related to my research and, as one of them was with my husband, I don't think that one really counts. One solitary moment of transcendence, then. (If Ben had been able to keep Dominic occupied for another hour on the night I met Sebastian, who knows, it could have been two.) To think of all the money I've spent getting one singular sensation. I could have bought a power shower for a quarter of the price.

Months and months of treating sex as a non-contact sport had rubbed off in my bedroom. I did say 'yes' to Dominic on occasion but only when he tipped my head forward first. I had become the type of woman who, after much coaxing, would agree to lifting up her nightie for five minutes, but only with the light out. Ben said he was planning to go out and buy a nightie so he could be like it too. We had become erotically challenged.

If, after reading this book, you still don't understand the eroticism around sexual infantilism or adult boarding schools, or any of the other things I've done, then join the club. I entered into these activities (or sent Ben in my place) because I wanted to know how it felt. At the Muir Reform Academy, I felt like a thirty-four-year-old woman in an ill-fitting school uniform. At the Hush-A-Bye-Baby Club, Ben felt like a complete idiot. Neither of us had the desire to feel like school children or babies. And what's sex without desire?

Thinking of England? Thinking of Emigrating.

Encyclopedia of Unusual Sexual Practices

Brenda Love

Some people have sex with armpits. Honestly. And, as Brenda Love explains in this extraordinary book, there's even a name for it: axillism.

Axillism is just one of hundreds of activities explored in the *Encyclopedia of Unusual Sex Practices*, a truly mind-boggling guide to the enormous diversity of human sexual expression. From the mildly kinky to the downright bizarre (not to say painful), the *Encyclopedia* lists all the forms of arousal you can imagine, and many more you can't.

A mere sample of this sexual smorgasbord reveals such gems as 'queening' (woman sitting on man's head); 'dogging' (sex in parked cars); 'felching' (look it up) and pyrophilia (don't even think about it).

Whatever turns you on, this book will have it. Whether for handy reference or general interest, the *Encyclopedia of Unusual Sex Practices* makes for stimulating and absolutely fascinating reading.

'*Will fill you with astonishment at the inventiveness of human beings in pursuit of pleasure and novelty*' – Isadora Alman, Village Voice

Abacus
0 349 10676 2

Sex in History

Reay Tannahill

Sex in History chronicles the pleasures – and the perils – of the flesh from the time of mankind's distant ancestors to the modern day; from a sexual act which was brief, crude and purposeful, to the myriad varieties of contemporary sexual mores.

Reay Tannahill's accessible study ranges from the earliest forms of contraception (one Egyptian concoction included crocodile dung) to some latter-day misconceptions about it – like the men who joined their lovers in taking the Pill 'just to be on the safe side'. It surveys all manner of sexual practice, preference and position (the acrobatic 'wheelbarrow' position, the strenuous 'hovering butterflies' position . . .) and draws on sources as diverse as the *Admirable Discourses of the Plain Girl*, the *Exhibition of Female Flagellants, Important Matters of the Jade Chamber* and *The Romance of Chastisement*.

Whether writing on androgyny, courtly love, flagellation or zoophilia, Turkish eunuchs, Greek dildoes, Taoist sex manuals or Japanese geisha girls, Reay Tannahill is consistently enlightening and entertaining.

'*Level-headed . . . diligent, provocative and fascinating. The book is the most complete of its kind ever written*' – Time

'*Sanity on the subject of sex is all too rare; wit is in even shorter supply and an engaging style is about as commonplace as eyebrows on an egg. Three cheers, therefore, for Reay Tannahill*' – Washington Post

Abacus
0 349 10486 7

Up North

Charles Jennings

The North.

Where does it begin? Were does it end? And is it all whippets, black pudding, and queer folk going round saying 'There's nowt so queer as folk'?

Fresh from the P.J. O'Rourke School of Diplomatic Journalism, southern jessie Charles Jennings finds himself in need of Answers. With something approaching trepidation, Jennings packs his big girl's blouse in a suitcase full of prejudice and ventures fearfully into the great melting-pot that is the North of England – undergoing in the process a series of life-changing experiences such as being mistaken for an exhibit at the *Wigan Pier: Where History Comes Alive!* museum and voluntarily attending a concert featuring Roy Walker.

Scandalous, astonishingly rude, scabrously funny, *Up North* presents the quintessential northern experience.

'*Jennings is blessed with a tremendous sense of humour and a gift for piercingly evocative prose . . . blissfully funny*' – Sunday Telegraph

'*We can laugh off most of the drivel spoken by self-opinionated political commentators and comedians, but Mr Jennings has gone too far*' – John Towndrow, mayor of Scunthorpe

'*Like Orwell, Jennings has an unerring eye for tat and bright-eyed failure . . . Very funny, appalled and unbelieving*' – New Statesman

Abacus
0 349 10685 1

Generation X

Douglas Coupland

Andy, Dag and Claire have been handed a society priced beyond their means. Twentysomethings, brought up with divorce, Watergate and Three Mile Island, and scarred by the 80s fall-out of yuppies, recession, crack and Ronald Reagan, they represent the new lost generation – Generation X.

Fiercely suspicious of being lumped together as an advertiser's target market, they have quit dreary careers and cut themselves adrift in the California desert; in Palm Springs, land of the liposuction clinic and the shopping mall, dumping-ground for the dregs of American cultural memory.

Unsure of their futures, they immerse themselves in a regime of heavy drinking and working at McJobs – 'low-pay, low-prestige, low-benefit, no-future jobs in the service industry'. Underemployed, overeducated, intensely private and unpredictable, they have nowhere to direct their anger, no one to assuage their fears, and no culture to replace their anomie. So they tell stories; disturbingly funny tales that reveal their barricaded inner world. A world populated with dead TV show, 'Elvis moments' and semi-disposable Swedish furniture . . .

'*Funny, colourful and accessible, this is a blazing début*' – The Times

'*Riotous . . . truly a modern-day* Catcher in the Rye' – Cosmopolitan

'*Quirky, witty, with an affection for its characters which lifts it above the level of such as Bret Easton Ellis's* Less Than Zero' – Mail on Sunday

'*The overall effect is something close to a New Age J.D. Salinger on smart drugs*' – Time Out

'*Fiercely comic*' – Sunday Express

Abacus
0 349 10331 3

☐ ENCYCLOPEDIA OF UNUSUAL SEX PRACTICES	Brenda Love	£12.99
☐ SEX IN HISTORY	Reay Tannahill	£9.99
☐ UP NORTH	Charles Jennings	£6.99
☐ GENERATION X	Douglas Coupland	£6.99

Abacus now offers an exciting range of quality titles by both established and new authors which can be ordered from the following address:

Little, Brown and Company (UK),
P.O. Box 11,
Falmouth,
Cornwall TR10 9EN.

Fax No: 01326 317444
Telephone No: 01326 317200
E-mail: books@barni.avel.co.uk

Payments can be made as follows: cheque, postal order (payable to Little, Brown and Company) or by credit cards, Visa/Access. Do not send cash or currency. UK customers and B.F.P.O. please allow £1.00 for postage and packing for the first book, plus 50p for the second book, plus 30p for each additional book up to a maximum charge of £3.00 (7 books plus).

Overseas customers including Ireland please allow £2.00 for the first book plus £1.00 for the second book, plus 50p for each additional book.

NAME (block letters) ....

....

ADDRESS ....

....

....

☐ I enclose my remittance for _____

☐ I wish to pay by Access/Visa card

Number ☐☐☐☐☐☐☐☐☐☐☐☐☐☐☐☐☐☐

Card Expiry Date ☐☐☐☐